The
Roses
Speak

The
Roses
Speak

A Chronic Illness
Journey

James Menkhaus

NCP
NEW CITY PRESS

Published in the United States by New City Press
136 Madison Avenue, Floors 5 & 6, PMB #4290
New York, NY 10016
www.newcitypress.com

The Roses Speak
A Chronic Illness Journey

Cover design and layout by Miguel Tejerina

Library of Congress Cataloging-in-Publication Data
Library of Congress Control Number: 2024953095
ISBN: 978-1-56548-649-2 (paper)
ISBN: 978-1-56548-666-9 (e-book)

Printed in Canada

To the cystic fibrosis community:
May we never cease to share our stories.
Roses make the world more beautiful.

When the Roses Speak, I Pay Attention

"As long as we are able to
be extravagant we will be
hugely and damply
extravagant. Then we will drop
foil by foil to the ground. This
is our unalterable task, and we do it
joyfully."

And they went on, "Listen,
the heart-shackles are not, as you think,
death, illness, pain,
unrequited hope, not loneliness, but

lassitude, rue, vainglory, fear, anxiety,
selfishness."

Their fragrance all the while rising
from their blind bodies, making me
spin with joy.

—Mary Oliver

Contents

Preface

Discovering My Truth

My father drove me to school each morning during my first year of high school. Traveling in his brown Chevy pickup truck, from the west side of Cincinnati to St. Xavier, took approximately thirty minutes, leaving ample time for father-son life discussions. One morning, I pulled out the most recent edition of *Blueprint*, the school newspaper, which I had hastily thrown into my backpack the previous day. I expected to read the headlines out loud and share the latest school news. As my eyes scanned the front page, I became silent. It felt like a pit in my stomach, and my heart began to race. I was unable to speak as my eyes darted across the page.

Bold letters splashed across the front stating, "Luedeke Battles CF." The article revealed that Mr. Andrew Luedeke, a faculty member at St. Xavier, received a double lung transplant within the past three years because he had cystic fibrosis (CF). Although he had been healthy enough to teach following the transplant, scar tissue developed on his lungs, and he was going to require another transplant to stay alive. The teachers quoted in the article did not sound optimistic about his recovery. One faculty member acknowledged that even being alive in his late twenties made Luedeke "a walking miracle." Another stated, "Most young people die from cystic fibrosis in their mid-twenties. Andy is in his mid-thirties. He's beaten a lot of odds."[1] I reread that sentence over and over, making sure I saw it correctly. My body froze. A chill ran down my spine. I flipped back to the front page to a box with facts on cystic fibrosis. The box read, "Median Survival: 29 years."

---

1.   Andy Amend, "Luedeke Battles CF," *Blueprint,* March 1, 1996.

I looked toward my father, struggling to find the words I wanted to say to him. "There is a teacher at St. X . . . who has CF. They think he is going to die." My father remained silent. "And it says here that the life expectancy is twenty-nine. That means . . . I have already lived half my life." I was processing these words as I spoke. My father quietly replied, "You never know about those things. You could live a long time." He choked up as he struggled to find a way to support his son who, for the first time, learned that his disease was terminal. For the rest of the day, I was in a trance, going from class to class and occasionally rereading the article. A deep sadness tinged with fear overtook me. I was overwhelmed by the unfairness that I would not get to live as long as my classmates who sat beside me. I felt heavy, moving through the day as if I was stuck in quicksand. The day seemed twice as long as any other, and I just wanted to go home to cry. Each time I pulled the paper from my backpack, it did not change: "Median Survival: 29 years."

I still remember how I felt reading that newspaper article. I was shocked, afraid, and then felt powerless. That day was the start of a new chapter of my life that dramatically altered how I saw myself, the world, and my future. Two years after reading that headline, I began to develop lung complications, which is one of the more common manifestations of CF. Mucus in my lungs began to slowly destroy the airways. My new and constant coughing was an ever-present reminder of Mr. Luedeke and his need for a lung transplant to extend his life.

Following high school, I moved to Cleveland, Ohio to attend John Carroll University. My new treatment regimen went with me. Luckily, a new advancement for fighting CF had recently become available. It was a vest that would shake a person, causing the mucus to dislodge from the airways so it could be expelled. I also used multiple inhalers while doing these vest treatments to make coughing up the secretions easier on my lungs and muscles. These treatments took an hour each day and kept me relatively healthy during my time in college. However, facing a constant battle to stay alive and completing daily treatments in my dorm made me feel very alone.

By the time I graduated college, my lung issues resulted in a steady stream of inpatient hospital treatments and IV PICC lines[2] to stave off the infections that were slowly killing my lungs. I was losing 3–5% of my lung function per year. Despite being active and adhering to the myriad treatments for fifteen years, by 2019 I found myself meeting with doctors to discuss a lung transplant. As I left that meeting, I thought of Mr. Luedeke. My CF experience was coming full circle. As a high school student, I learned the truly precarious nature of having CF from a newspaper article. Now, I would consider the procedure that gave Mr. Luedeke a few extra years of life before he died.

On January 1, 2020, however, my decline took a dramatic detour. That morning, I took my first dose of Trikafta. Within twenty-four hours, my body began to change. My constant coughing decreased and eventually disappeared. I experienced strength and energy that I had not felt for a long time. I did not realize it then, but that day began a new phase of my life. Nearly twenty-five years after reading the headline in my high school newspaper, I was once again overtaken by emotions and overwhelmed by intense feelings. However, this time it was not about decreased life expectancy, but about a previously unimaginable possibility of a longer, healthier life. In the weeks following my first dose, I saw vast improvements in my stamina. I began to gain weight for the first time since middle school.[3] I eagerly mused about the possibilities for my future.

As I began to embrace this optimism, the specter of COVID-19 overshadowed everything, and lockdowns became a way of life. People around the world feared for their own survival. Especially for those living with a lung disease, 2020 was a frightening time to

---

2. Peripherally Inserted Central Catheter (PICC) lines are often inserted in the arm and are advanced to a large central vein near the heart. They are used for long-term IV antibiotic medications.
3. Gaining weight can be especially difficult for those with CF due to malabsorption. Thick mucus can clog the pancreatic ducts, leading to impaired delivery of enzymes and poor uptake of nutrients. People with CF often experience increased energy needs due to infections and increased efforts to breathe while having a decreased appetite.

be alive. Headlines that could have been about CF patients having new opportunities in life were displaced by warnings of an illness killing people every day. I didn't take the time to process what was happening inside of me because there was so much to process outside of me.

I believed at age fifteen that I had lived half my life. I learned that I was going to die. Trikafta has given me a reprieve and extended my life expectancy, but I still live with CF every day. Coming to terms with death is not only a reality for those with cystic fibrosis. Death is the one experience that every human person has in common. Mortality can be a scary realization. It certainly was for me as a teenager. However, a median survival age doesn't define who I am. This book will give insight into the ways having a chronic illness can affect a person. It is an invitation for all people to reflect on mortality and the fragility of existence. This is not only a CF story. It is the human story.

Acknowledgments

This book would not exist without the honesty and vulnerability of the people whose stories you will encounter. I am grateful to those with cystic fibrosis who shared their story with me: Riley Aroche, Morgan Barrett, Grace-Rose Bauer, Ryne Beck, Hilary Becker, Mark Bettinger, Malik Bishop, Emma Boniface, Devin Broadbent, Annabelle Brown, Casey Bruce, Jerry Cahill, Eliza Callard, Erika Castrucci, Talia Cestone, Alexa Ciancimino, Will Corcoran, Maddie Core, Marc Cotterill, Erica Daley, Jaime Dunaway, Teresa Dunning, Tyler Engle, Marina Finnell, Adrian Flor, Justin Goldsmith, Raelene Goody, Lyndall Grace, Caleigh Haber, Steph Hansen, Chase Honeycutt, Anissa Hostetter, Molly Jensen, Kassandra Klemenz, Emily Kramer-Golinkoff, Nick Laing, Jarrod Landau, Emily Lawrence, Andy Lipman, Andrii Lukianets, Debra Mattson, Erin McCaw, Ryann McCoy, Brian McTear, Rachel Meddaugh, Brandon Miller, Joshua Mitchell, Pat Mitchell, Haley Moreland, Beth Morgan, Dylan Mortimer, Ben Mudge, Becca Mueller, Cheri Nel, Maude Perrine, Sonja Petrovic, Jess Pickering, Tricia Polzin, Jess Ragusa, Dugan Reilly, Monique Renee, Adem Riahi, James Richardson, Helen Roper, Kari Rose, Katherine Russell, Rachael Russell, Emily Schaller, McKenzie Schneider, Kathleen Schwartz, Pug Scoville, Sarah Skeffington, Andy Smith, Martin Smith, Reid Jewett Smith, Travis Suit, Zack Swanborn, Martin Tallant, Kira Taylor, Clark Thiemann, Darren Turner, Eric Verdon, Rylee Walker, Stephen Walter, Bryan Warnecke, Tess Weber, Lori White, Lizzie Whitla, Mason Williams, Bonnie-Rose Wise, and Justyna Zaskwara.

I am equally grateful to those who shared stories about their loved ones, both living and deceased, with cystic fibrosis: Brynn Baskin (uncle Bruce Baskin), Laura Bonnell (daughters Emily and Molly Bonnell), Victoria DiSorbo (friend Julie), Marcos Gonzales (nephew Xavier Guerrero), Liz Hammel (daughter Maeve Hammel), Pat Mitchell (great-grandson Hudson Parker), Collette Portner (daughter Ravyn Gabel), Shwetha Sree (son Vihaan Krishna), Candace Taylor (daughter Isla Taylor), Paula van Wyk (son Jack

Peck), Beth Vanstone (daughter Madi Vanstone), and Ashley Williams (daughter Aurora Mcarter).

I also spoke with current or former members of CF care teams to have a greater understanding of how CF care has changed over time, and I am grateful to: Theresa Frantzen, Denis Hadjiliadis, Rosa Mascola, Casey McCullough, Angela Oder, and Katherine Papia for sharing their insights and expertise.

Writing this book occurred predominantly while I was engaged in Clinical Pastoral Education (CPE) training as a hospital chaplain. I am grateful to my Cleveland Clinic CPE internship group of Stephen Ntui, Diane Rhynes, Natalie Kertesz, and educators, Bob McGeeney and Jim Egolf, for helping me begin to process my own health journey. My one-year residency at Covenant Healthcare, in Saginaw, Michigan, guided me in further exploration of my life. The support of my CPE residency group, Henry Adesiji, Amy Dobyns, Jeremy Lobdell, educator Ron Cooper, and Kathy Bonn, the director of the Pastoral Care Department, was invaluable. CPE was a challenging and beautiful gift that invited me to examine my story while I accompanied others exploring their own.

Many people read drafts of this manuscript and offered helpful suggestions and ideas. I am grateful to Eric Abercrombie, Jeff Bloodworth, Nicole Bubie, Sean Cahill, Samantha Cocco, Ron Cooper, Paula Fitzgerald, Paul Lauritzen, Rosa Mascola, Michael Moore, and Katlyn Unger for their time and insight. The initial research for the book began as an independent study course with Maggie Hatch and Clara Morgan, who helped me think through the interview process. Maggie, Rachel Schratz, and Rylee Walker became a team that helped me with research, brainstorming, and editing throughout the project. I am very thankful for their constant help, support, and encouragement.

I would not be alive today without the love and support of my parents, Ed and Carol, who had no experience raising a child with a chronic illness. They always supported me in every way possible. I am also grateful for the friends in my life who have buoyed me through times of struggle and illness. Finally, this publication would not be possible without the staff at New City Press. Thank you for making it possible for everyone to hear the roses speak.

Introduction

The Extravagance of Storytelling

Dear Diary, I am holding back tears of joy as I write this entry. It's the second day of my high school Kairos retreat. Tonight, I did something I never thought I would do. I had an opportunity to share my story in front of my classmates, and I could feel something inside of me pulling me to stand up. You know how shy I am. Suddenly, I was walking toward the front of the room. It was like my feet had a mind of their own! My heart was pumping so fast. As I approached the podium, I looked out at everyone staring at me. I cleared my throat and began speaking. "My name is Jimmy . . . and . . . I have cystic fibrosis. . . . I want to share my story."

Cystic fibrosis is an inherited genetic disease affecting over 105,000 people across ninety-four countries. Nearly 40,000 of those people live in the United States.[4] As a chronic and terminal illness, there is currently no cure. Cystic fibrosis shares this designation with cancer, multiple sclerosis, Parkinson's disease, AIDS, and many other incurable conditions. Each of these illnesses has unique and debilitating aspects that can make life challenging, difficult, and painful for those with the disease as well as those supporting

---

4. "About Cystic Fibrosis." *Cystic Fibrosis Foundation*, https://www.cff.org/intro-cf/about-cystic-fibrosis.

them. In the case of many chronic illnesses, those afflicted can find themselves marginalized by the greater population. They may face legal and medical barriers to their care and come to feel they are more of a burden than a person worthy of love and support. They may also feel alone, especially when their condition causes them to endure hardships that no one around them can conceptualize. While this book will focus predominantly on the experiences of those living and dying within the CF community, I hope that people with other conditions will come to discover some of their own story in these pages.

Sixty-Five Roses

Charlie Fry wasn't always a "boy wonder" from the UK. In fact, he wasn't great at football, or as it is known in the US, soccer. His poor lungs held him back. "It made it hard for him to breathe—and he was never hungry. He had to do physiotherapy each day and take a lot of medicine too. If he got ill though, it almost always meant . . . a two-week hospital stay."[5] While walking home one day after a game, he was struck by lightning. Suddenly everything went blank. He woke up in the hospital with a new skill. He saw a target that helped him guide the ball into the goal. Instead of being bullied for his sickly demeanor, Charlie became the star of his team. He still struggled with his chronic-illness identity, wondering why he couldn't be like everyone else.[6] However, he had something that gave him strength and helped him cope. It was the beginning of his self-discovery as an eleven-year-old boy.

Charlie Fry isn't a real person. He is a fictional character in a children's book created by Martin Smith. Martin is in his mid-forties, lives in the UK, and has cystic fibrosis. Unlike Charlie, Martin is not a football star. He was a journalist for fifteen years before his health declined. He began coughing up so much blood

---

5. Martin Smith, *The Football Boy Wonder: The Charlie Fry Series* (Create Space Independent Publishing Platform, 2015), 15.
6. Smith, *Football Boy Wonder*, 105.

that he was unable to work.[7] No longer healthy enough to continue in journalism, in 2014 he applied his writing skills to a new genre—children's books. Charlie Fry, whose initials are CF, was born. "Everyone who reads it gets a little bit of understanding about cystic fibrosis," Martin explained. Charlie's diagnosis represents more than a reflection of Martin's life living with a chronic illness. It makes a statement about the importance of having a main character who achieves despite a chronic illness. "How often do you see a character in a book or TV series that isn't able-bodied? It rarely happens," Martin expressed. He has been blown away by the support of parents of children with CF who have written to him to tell him how much their children enjoy the series. Charlie represents the challenges of living with a chronic illness, inviting readers to reflect on the ways there may be some of Charlie in all of us.

Although Charlie Fry is fictional, the way Martin describes the life of a person with CF is accurate for some people. There are many nuances to having cystic fibrosis and there is only one thing that is common among all people with CF. People who genetically inherit two copies of a mutated cystic fibrosis transmembrane conductance regulator (CFTR) gene will have cystic fibrosis.[8] Beyond biology, one can speak of common CF indicators, but the disease can vary widely from person to person. Most people with CF experience lung issues caused by the buildup of mucus. This mucus destroys the lung airways, potentially resulting in the need for a lung transplant, like Mr. Luedeke. Many people also have degenerative destruction to their pancreas, which interferes with food digestion and can lead to type 1 diabetes. Other gastrointestinal complications can lead to liver, kidney, and/or stomach issues.

---

7. Coughing up blood is known as hemoptysis. It is a common progression of CF due to infection and/or irritation of the pulmonary blood vessels that can cause them to become more delicate over time.

8. "Cystic Fibrosis Causes," *National Heart, Lung, and Blood Institute* (NIH), https://www.nhlbi.nih.gov/health/cystic-fibrosis/causes#:~:text=Cystic%20fibrosis%20is%20an%20inherited,parent)%20will%20have%20cystic%20fibrosis

A person may have any combination of these symptoms in varying degrees. It is also important to know that there are different genetic mutations, which affect treatment. What might work with one group may not work with another.[9]

The treatment disparity based on gene type became heightened with the advent of gene modulators. These treatments are not antibiotics. These medications modulate the CFTR genes. The most recent and successful modulator, Trikafta, has split CF into camps of those who benefit from it and those who do not. The group who has not had their lives changed by Trikafta can be broken into three distinct groups: those who do not have access, those whose gene type prohibits it from working, and those who have access and the operative gene type, but experienced side effects that prevent it from being a viable option. All these categories will be represented in this book through people's stories.

Cystic fibrosis manifestations vary so widely that it is possible for a person to test positive for CF later in life (or never) and to have lived with no outward signs. Pug Scoville, from Florida, was diagnosed at the age of seventy-two. He was being treated for bronchiectasis when one of his doctors decided to test if he had CF because he would cough for thirty to forty minutes each night. "It got to the point where I dreaded going to bed," he recalled. To his surprise, the results were positive for CF. Pug faces unique challenges living with CF in his seventies. For example, he has a pacemaker, and using his therapy vest increases his heart rate and gives him chest pains. "This was the first time somebody with a pacemaker was also using a SmartVest," he explained. After unsuccessful attempts to modify his pacemaker, doctors recommended other forms of airway clearance. Pug also explained that Medicare doesn't give the same financial assistance as other insurers for Trikafta. Luckily, a recent Medicare provision caps

---

9. "Types of CF Mutations," *Cystic Fibrosis Foundation*, https://www.cff.org/research-clinical-trials/types-cftr-mutations#:~:text=There%20are%20five%20classes%20of,different%20types%20of%20CFTR%20mutations. There are five major classes of CFTR proteins.

the out-of-pocket maximum for drug prescriptions, making it more affordable. Few people have lived to Pug's age with CF, so funding for Trikafta is a new frontier. He is paving the way for a future where more people live into their seventies.

Because CF can be so devastating, it is difficult for many to imagine living seventy years. Malik Bishop, who lives in Houston, Texas, felt the effects of having CF before he was aware of the world. He was diagnosed at birth and quickly put into a foster home. "I had CF, and my parents weren't . . . equipped to handle that because they were just out of high school," he reflected. Malik considered his disease "moderate" growing up. "I didn't really notice much difference between me and the other kids until I was in the third or fourth grade," Malik recalled. During sports, he would stop to use his inhaler, just as Martin Smith described with the fictional Charlie Fry. To date, Malik's form of CF has focused more on gastrointestinal complications than lung issues, while he contends with constant bouts of pneumonia, weight loss, and mental health challenges. Like some people you will meet in this book, Trikafta has been life-changing for Malik. "It was . . . the difference between night and day since the very first dose," he emotionally shared.

You will read the stories of many people with CF, like Pug and Malik. I invite you to imagine each speaker as a rose, and as the title of the Mary Oliver poem instructs, when the roses speak, pay attention. The rose image is not my own but derives from the story of four-year-old Ricky Weiss. Ricky heard his mother describing fundraising to help find a cure for her son's illness. Ricky heard "cystic fibrosis" and pronounced it "sixty-five roses." Since 1965, "sixty-five roses" has represented CF.[10] Thus, the title of this book combines the image of the rose with the importance of hearing the story told by the chronically ill themselves. I allude to Mary Oliver's poem throughout the book because it tells the tale of the roses who speak truths about what is important in life before

---

10. "65 Roses Story," *Cystic Fibrosis Foundation*, https://www.cff.org/about-us/65-roses-story.

falling to the ground in death. I hope you find the wisdom of the roses in this book—insights from those who have navigated life acutely aware they are dying.

Sometimes stories are told better without words. Dylan Mortimer, from Kansas City, communicates his CF story through images. He loved art since he was eight years old, which inspired his pursuit of art degrees in college and graduate school. In 2017, when Dylan's health began to fail rapidly, he needed his first lung transplant. Two years later, he needed a second transplant and received a new set of lungs. Dylan explained, "Receiving lungs is a gift that takes you out of yourself, it is very humbling." Following his first transplant, Dylan felt a desire to connect his health issues with his artistic gifts. "It felt dishonest to not bring it in in some way," he explained.

Dylan's artwork now hangs in hospitals and clinics around the country. He feels this is a way to bring inspiration to places where people most need it. He also collaborates with *CF Vests Worldwide*, a nonprofit organization that works to donate therapy vests to people in countries where they may not have access to this lifesaving equipment. When a person is sent a vest, they receive some of Dylan's artwork, which he hopes is a way to combine the "physical aim with a sort of metaphysical inspiration and hope." Dylan hopes that his art will be a "way to engage people, . . . spread awareness, and invite other people into [his] story, . . . [by] connecting [it] to their story and creating community." Dylan's narrative doesn't use words. But it tells his story.

Transformative stories can also be expressed through music. Brian McTear lives in Philadelphia, where he is a music producer, writer, and singer. He runs a widely respected recording studio called *Miner Street Recordings* and a music nonprofit called *Weathervane Music*. The mission of *Weathervane Music* is to advance independent music, art, and the communities around those who create this music. On December 6, 2019, he played his own songs at a holiday concert. Three days earlier, he began taking Trikafta. This concert was his chance for his mother and friends to hear him sing with clear lungs. "The ability to sing in that concert I had not experienced in fifteen years," he reflected. "The clarity of my breathing [was] pristine. It was virtually overnight," he explained about the hours following his first dose. The name of his first song from that concert was "You paralyze my heart." One can only imagine how his loved ones were paralyzed in shock hearing Brian's new voice, as his unparalyzed lungs were filling and exhaling. What a gift for Brian to be able to sing for his mother, who was sitting in the front row on such a beautiful occasion. Brian's CF story isn't told as a written narrative. It is poetry put to music; the song of new life offered in a community of love.

Music may also provide a metaphor for how to read this book. Different vocal ranges, such as tenor, bass, alto, and soprano, come together to form a harmonious sound. Sometimes these voices seem to be communicating a different message, such as when a choir utilizes polyphony—simultaneously singing different lines. The goal of this technique is not to sound dissonant, but to bring out different aspects of the song. In the same way, people with CF may have very different experiences. The voices may not "sound" the same, and it may be difficult to fathom that they have the same medical condition. However, when hearing the voices communicate together, you will realize their harmony and a united message of singing for the day when CF stands for "cure found."

The Roses Speak is the combined story of many members of the CF community, a glimpse into the world of a chronic illness. It is a representation of people who may feel silenced or ignored because their medical conditions may impair their lives. I am not trying to tell *the* CF story. I am trying to tell CF stories. I invite those with conditions other than CF to see how their journey has similarities to this CF narrative. No one can tell another person's story. No one can truly know what someone else is going through. The best we can do is offer our own story to another and create an environment for storytelling. When that happens, it can be a powerful moment where we come to see the Charlie Fry in each of us.

Data with a Soul

A way to conceptualize the layout of the book is to think of your favorite movie. If someone watched twenty minutes of the climactic sequence, but not the final ten minutes of the movie, it would feel incomplete. You might see the most action-packed part or the big reveal of a mystery, but you would have no idea who the characters are, why the issue exists, or how it concludes. Yes, Trikafta has become a miraculous medication that has saved and transformed lives. It has certainly extended my life far beyond what I expected. However, a fuller picture is needed to appreciate and understand the story of CF in the gene modulator era. Plot, action, and characters develop within a setting and a history. I intend this book to give insight into the "before" and "after" of Trikafta, not just the miraculous present. Appreciating a butterfly is even more amazing when viewed next to a caterpillar.

For those interested in understanding the historical development of CF treatment from the discovery of the CF gene through the early days of gene modulators, I highly recommend *Breath from Salt*, by Bijal Trivedi. Although she does not have CF, Trivedi's well-researched work beautifully tells of the discovery of CF and the vast efforts at care development and fundraising that make gene modulators possible. *The Roses Speak* serves as a continuation of her work. I have chosen to spend less time on historical aspects of CF and CF treatment, as I think *Breath from Salt* has given that to the CF community. *The Roses Speak* focuses more on the psychological, emotional, and spiritual journey told through the eyes of those with CF.

To tell these stories, I needed to find people willing to share, while reflecting on my own story. The method for this research began by emailing more than one hundred directors of CF clinics in the United States. I received roughly thirty responses, with most centers agreeing to advertise in their newsletter. The *CF Foundation* also sent an invitation to their LISTSERV. About 20 percent of the people interviewed came from these two approaches. Around 70 percent of respondents came from the 400 people

I reached out to over *Instagram* who used a CF-related hashtag. The other 10 percent came from personal invitations to others by people who had been interviewed. These interviews occurred virtually, between February 2023 and October 2024.

I never expected how powerful these conversations would be for me. What began as research into CF and Trikafta became research into myself. As people shared stories and created spaces for vulnerability, I found myself sharing my own. I can't recall a single interview where something did not touch my own story. I had only spoken to one person with CF in my life prior to this project. Other people articulated the same form of loneliness. Researching and writing this book were gifts for me; I hope reading it is a gift for you.

During the fifteen months of writing, I was an intern and resident in clinical pastoral education (CPE). My internship was at the Cleveland Clinic, during the summer of 2023, and my residency was at Covenant Healthcare, in Saginaw, Michigan, from September 2023 to August 2024. CPE involves training as a hospital chaplain, sitting with the sick and dying, and hearing their stories. By being present in these times of vulnerability, a chaplain listens for a patient's primary unmet spiritual needs, such as fear when learning a new prognosis, loneliness and isolation, and presence during grief. Once identified, a chaplain attempts interventions, such as guidance in decision-making, reconciliation with others, or finding value in themselves.[11] I found this application for theology incredibly powerful, since I had previously taught theology. A CPE student also spends one day a week in a classroom exploring one's own story and learning tools for pastoral accompaniment. Unlike in movies, chaplains do more than pray with patients. While prayer certainly happens, chaplains also can help a patient explore their innermost feelings and motivations.

---

11. Michele Shields, Allison Kastenbaum, and Laura B. Dunn, "Spiritual AIM and the Work of the Chaplain: A Model for Assessing Spiritual Needs and Outcomes in Relationships," in *Palliative Support Care* (2015, 13:1), 75–89.

The level of religiosity is entirely up to the patient and the family. Hospital chaplains do not convert or proselytize. They accompany people on the journey of life and help them explore their own stories.[12]

I am very grateful that I was writing this book while learning in CPE. CPE gave me tools to recognize how the CF discussions touched my own story. I grew in my understanding of the importance of listening through the healthcare setting, helping patients to feel seen and heard through the cultivation of skills such as wondering, following, and holding. In *See Me as a Person*, one of the texts used in our CPE training, authors Mary Koloroutis and Michael Trout write, "[Stories] are ways to interpret the past and to be intentional about the future. They can help us move beyond our simple cognitive thinking into accessing our emotional feelings about situations, which can then lead us to new insights and deepen our understanding."[13]

Koloroutis and Trout cite author Brené Brown, who writes, "stories are data with a soul." Another way of conceptualizing this book is through Brown's image. Yes, it is research, and I hope it contributes to the accompaniment and caregiving toward those with chronic conditions. It is also more than research. The "data" you will read is the unfolding narrative of those who have lived with a chronic illness and how these stories are embodied by the individual's way of "wondering, following, and holding" the experience. The Latin word for soul is *anima*, from which we get the English word "animation." When a cartoon is animated, it comes alive, jumping off the page. I suspect there will be moments when this data jumps off the page and, in connecting to your story, jumps into your heart.

---

12. To protect patient rights and adhere to HIPAA, stories from my chaplain experience will not contain specific names, ages, diagnoses, or identifying information about patients or family members. Some minor details may be changed as well.

13. Mary Koloroutis and Michael Trout, *See Me as a Person: Creating Therapeutic Relationships* (Creative Healthcare Management, 2012), 20.

At one of my early visits during chaplain residency, I sat with a family of children in their thirties as their mother was dying of complications of cancer and lung failure. Her family asked me to say a few words to her about the afterlife, to "reassure" her in her faith. They explained that their mother, a devout Catholic, had voiced fears the previous night concerning where she would go after her death. As my intervention, I shared words of consolation about God's love, drawing upon her Catholic tradition. She appeared able to hear me as she struggled for breath. She died a few hours later. When I was called to her room, her family asked me to offer a prayer. We gathered around her bedside, held hands, and prayed. We then sat and I invited them to share a story about her as a way to begin their grief processing. What followed was laughing, crying, and storytelling, as they remembered how much she supported each of them in her own loving way. With tears rolling down her cheeks, the daughter nearest me expressed, "I never knew sharing stories about my mother with a complete stranger could be so cathartic." Her observation beautifully encapsulated one way to deal with grief and loss and has stayed with me as one of the more powerful moments of my development as a chaplain. Those stories also helped me reflect on my life, my relationship with my mother, and the empathy I felt toward this family. Their stories were cathartic for me as well.

I hope that the sharing of stories for this book was as helpful to those who told them, as it will be to those who will hear them. I hope you will see, hear, and feel some of your own humanity, vulnerability, and fragility. Perhaps the roses will increase your empathy toward those with a chronic disease or those who are experiencing the debilitating reality of old age. Maybe you will experience hope hearing stories of the miraculous, or you might realize you are not alone sitting with stories of sadness and loss. Finally, I hope this book encourages you to tell your story. No one else can. I describe, in the diary excerpt at the start of the Introduction, when I publicly shared for the first time that I had CF. While on that high school retreat, our leaders told us, "Boldly be yourself. There is only one of you for all time." Perhaps now I might amend the statement. Boldly tell your story. Only one person can tell it for all time.

Part One

Entering the Rose Garden

Living with a chronic illness can be an all-encompassing reality. Before discussing the transformative power of gene modulators, it is important to explore some of the ways people with CF, and many other chronic diseases, deal with illness every day. For some people, gene modulators have minimized CF symptoms, but these revolutionary medications are not cures. Taking one does not replace the gene that causes someone to have CF any more than being in remission means that someone does not have cancer. It means that a person *may* have a higher quality of life in the future. The longevity of the treatment is never assured. It is impossible to understand the potential of gene modulators without learning the reality of having CF without them.

I chose to start the book this way, rather than with the transformative power of gene modulators, for three reasons. First, most people with CF who take gene modulators continue to be affected by the psychology of how they lived prior to the medication. Second, it is impossible to appreciate the "miraculous" change of gene modulators, for good or bad, if you do not know what preceded this change. And third, there are people with CF who are not able to benefit from the current gene modulators for several reasons and still experience this as their predominant way of living with CF.

As you enter this rose garden, you will see a myriad of stories and experiences. As stated in the Introduction, there is not a singular CF story. While you peruse this rose garden, I hope you stop to admire the beauty of the roses. Take in the fragrance and admire the intricate uniqueness of each petal. Realize that scattered around are fallen petals, which dropped "foil by foil" to the ground. What might these roses teach about life from their perspective? How do they see the world differently? That is the "unalterable task" of Part One.

Chapter 1

The Greatest Lie Ever Told

I saw my first play tonight at St. Xavier. I don't remember the name of the play but, toward the end, the main character spoke about life and death. She said something about people not appreciating life while they live it. I was really struck by that line because . . . I don't think most people appreciate life. I got tears in my eyes when she said those lines. It was really embarrassing, and I did my best to make sure no one else saw that I was crying. I realize that no one in that room knows my secret, that I have CF and that I am dying. I know I don't have a lot of time to accomplish what I want to do with my life. I need to find out the name of the play so I can read it. Good night.

My encounter with the CF life expectancy through the school newspaper became a pivotal moment in my life. Chapter 1 illuminates how the prospect of a shortened lifespan may affect how a person with a chronic or terminal illness approaches time. I refer to this conceptualization of decreased life expectancy and slow degeneration of one's body as CF Time. This perspective is not exclusive to the cystic fibrosis community. People with other chronic or terminal conditions may also be able to relate to this experience. The observations about CF experiences should not be assumed to be universal in the CF or chronic illness communities. I only speak for myself and share what others have told me.

The Second Hand

When I began my first full-time job, I was asked by the human resources department if I would like to set aside a portion of my paycheck to begin contributing to my retirement. They explained that after the first year, it was mandatory; but during the first year, we had a choice if we wanted to invest or retain the money. There was little hesitation in my decision. "I'll take the money now," I responded. The human resources representative appeared shocked. That evening, I discussed this experience with a colleague. He, too, was surprised that I did not want to start investing in my retirement. He asked if I was planning to buy a house because, in the long-term, I would be wasting money if I rented an apartment. His advice was logical. But I was hearing it through the psychology of CF Time. My colleague had a family, a mortgage, and the anticipation of saving for his children's college fund. I had cystic fibrosis. At this time in my life, I calculated I had five years left until I would be too sick to work.

When I began this job, my FEV1[14] was in the low 60s[15] and had begun declining nearly 5% per year. I did not expect to live to the traditional retirement age. Forty years would be a gift and a shock. Sixty-five was unimaginable. I think my friend began to understand the gravity of living with CF following this conversation. Like many people, he knew CF was a serious condition but knew little about the specifics of living with it. I suspect being told by someone in his early thirties that he is expecting to only be healthy enough to work for a few years made it more tangible. As someone with no

---

14. FEV1 is the Forced Expiratory Volume (how much air you expel) in one second and is the primary value referenced by patients with CF. This is obtained from pulmonary function testing (PFT). PFTs are a series of tests that assess airflow, lung volume, and gas exchange signifying lung health, and are essential in monitoring disease progression. This is the number referred to as lung function.
15. 60% of what was predicted for a "normal" person my age, height, and gender. PFTs provide physical measurements along with a percent predicted that is based on the average expectation for a healthy person of similar age, weight, and gender.

spouse, no children, and no plan to be alive at sixty-five, I had no use for a retirement fund.

Grace-Rose Bauer, a college student studying film at New York University, describes growing up with a similar worldview. "When I was younger, I learned that having CF meant I may only live until around the age of ten. Psychologically, that messed me up," she recalled. Growing up with this knowledge would affect almost anyone, especially a child. "You kind of want to get everything done all at once; it all feels urgent," she acknowledged. Although she describes her health as less sick than many people with CF, growing up with the knowledge that "it was a progressive disease and could get worse and [she] could be in the hospital at any moment" greatly impacted her.

Despite these challenges, Grace-Rose credits her mother for always encouraging her to not let CF hold her back. "I am ten years past my expiration date at the moment," she asserted, as she was looking ahead to continuing her film studies. However, the lingering effects of growing up in CF Time still informs the way she processes her opportunities. "I think growing up with the idea that next year is never promised, I truly can't think far in advance," she admitted. When one of her friends told her, in 2023, that she was planning something for 2024, Grace-Rose had to tell her that she preferred not to make long-range plans. "It has something to do with being told growing up I didn't have long. This is a self-discovery I've recently realized," she mused. Such a view keeps her from contemplating too much about the future but can be motivating at the same time.

Grace-Rose captures what it is like to grow up with CF Time. Wrestling with universal realities like life and death can be hard for anyone. Imagine being ten and facing the reality of an imminent death. This can be especially confusing to a child who feels and appears healthy. Adding this developmental layer to the already difficult experience of growing up can be traumatizing. She explained that although her CF manifestations are not as severe as some, it is the possibility or likelihood that such a decline is both proximate and inevitable that makes it psychologically traumatizing. Being told decline is near, regardless of whether one feels sick, will radically affect how a young person views the potential future. One could become hopeless before the specter of the inevitable. To the usual skills of math, science, and spelling, and the rites of passage, like hormones and obtaining a driver's license, the young CF person adds breathing treatments, medications, hospital stays, and the psychological reality of a decreased mortality.

Having added responsibilities can force a CF child to grow up quickly. Molly Jensen, who recently graduated from high school, explained: "Learning how to navigate your disease at such a young age, being forced to be in tune with yourself . . . forces you to grow up a little faster." Like Grace-Rose, Molly found out about her life expectancy early in life. During a hospital visit, a genetic counselor told her, "I need you to start thinking about things in life based on your life expectancy." Molly was shocked to hear this as a twelve-year-old. She was told to pursue her passions early in life because "you never know how much time you will have to do that." "That conversation really hit me hard from the age of twelve to fifteen," Molly recalled. Echoing Grace-Rose, Molly explained how being constantly reminded of your life expectancy can have psychologically damaging effects. Realizing she couldn't put off doing things she enjoys, Molly became involved with therapy horse riding, which helped her to pursue her passion of being a horse trainer. She thoughtfully refers to this opportunity as "one of the biggest blessings of my life . . . because the other reality of 'I don't know if I will ever be able to do this' is so prevalent. It also makes the experiences in life I can do so much more meaningful."

CF Time may affect the choices a person makes and the way one understands time philosophically. One of the first times I recall reflecting on CF Time was in my teenage years while watching a scene in the movie *Star Trek: Generations*.[16] Watching *Star Trek* with my mother was one of the ways we bonded, and the show retains a special place in my heart. In the climactic scene, the villain Soran explains to Captain Picard his view on time. He defiantly states,

---

16. *Star Trek: Generations*, directed by David Carson (Paramount Pictures: 1994).

"We are all going to die sometime. It's just a question of how and when. You will too, Captain. Aren't you beginning to feel time gaining on you? It's like a predator. It's stalking you. Oh, you can try to outrun it with doctors, medicines, new technologies, but in the end, time is going to hunt you down and make the kill." Picard attempts a more positive spin by telling Soran that mortality is about the "truth of our existence" and is what defines humanity. I was quite taken by Soran's soliloquy. Since I had recently learned of Mr. Luedeke's illness, I had begun to contemplate my life expectancy, and the image of time as a stalker that was hunting me resonated.

A helpful image of life in CF Time is the difference between observing the hour hand and the second hand on a clock. One can stare at the hour hand and not detect its gradual movement. Intellectually, you know it is moving, but it is difficult to see. Most people without a health issue may approach time in this way. If you ask someone about life expectancy, they will likely say that life is short or precious, but most people rarely wake up every day thinking about time ticking down to their death. The hour hand moves slowly. Many people with a terminal illness, and those who are elderly, see life more like the second hand. The movement around the circle is obvious and ominous. You not only know it will work its way around, but you see it happening. As the popular phrase goes, seeing is believing. CF Time is the seeing of the second hand as it gets closer to its inevitable destination. The second hand is Soran's time predator preparing to move in for the kill.

My father's response when I told him about Mr. Luedeke was, "You never know, you could live a long time." This is certainly true. A chronic illness timeline is not a death sentence; however, growing up with this mentality, while slowly watching your body wither away in your teenage years or twenties, makes it *seem* an inevitable reality. Molly learned about her life expectancy through her genetic therapist during a hospital visit at the age of twelve. Many of the people I interviewed remembered learning their disease was terminal in their teens. Even the most hopeful person can easily become discouraged when last year they could climb stairs without stopping and the next year they get out of breath halfway up the stairs. If a doctor says it will only get worse, who am I to doubt what I feel *and* what I am told? This physical decline is likely to have a psychological impact.

Reid Jewett Smith is thirty-seven, a bit older than Grace-Rose and Molly. She also recalls living in CF Time and how that affected her life decisions. Six years ago, she began to pursue a PhD in education at Boston College. "This was sort of my swan song, and I expected to not be able to work again," she reflected, as her health was in decline. Unlike some who pursue graduate school for career advancement, Reid wanted to remove completing a doctorate from her bucket list. She never intended to use the degree. I felt the same way when I began my doctoral program at Duquesne University in 2007. I expected to be healthy enough to finish the program but never saw myself using the degree. Like Grace-Rose, the future was out of the realm of consideration.

Reid reflected that many decisions she took during her young adult life didn't really feel like they mattered. She enjoyed partying with friends and didn't think about the consequences of her actions. "It felt so low stakes. If I die at this college party from drinking too much or if I die five years later, . . . who cares? Every moment felt like YOLO [You Only Live Once]," she confided. It makes sense to live in the moment in CF Time because the moment is the only thing one can be sure exists. While this is not unique to people with a chronic illness, those with a shortened life expectancy are far more likely than the average person to die sooner. Life choices are weighted with a different calculus when you watch the second hand. Society tells people what they should want and how to be an adult. Those ground rules are pointless if the person believes they will never become an adult.

An analogy may help to elucidate this chronic illness declining mindset. Imagine your grandmother is widowed and in her late seventies. She is experiencing a decrease in mobility and mental faculties. One day you sit down to talk through the arrangements of transitioning her into a retirement home when your cousin says there are other options. This cousin thinks that despite her age, grandma could buy a new home, even though she is unable to clean and move around on her own. He also explains that grandma should begin to save money instead of spending it. She has always wanted to do another trip to Europe and in three to four years she will have set aside enough for the trip. She could also start a new career and make money that way. Finally, your cousin thinks grandma should begin online dating. Although she can no longer drive, there is no reason she can't "play the field" and potentially meet someone. "Life expectancy is just a number," your cousin optimistically proclaims.

This cousin has a good point about life expectancy. It is just a number. If grandma wants to go on a date or save money for something nice, these are not unreasonable possibilities. Her feelings and abilities can factor into these decisions. Other things, like buying a new home, planning to save for a trip to Europe, especially if she is already having mobility issues, and starting a new career, could be a bit more fanciful. Anyone who has had this type of care conversation with an aging loved one knows it is difficult to balance respect for autonomy, safety issues, and expressing appropriate expectations. These are difficult conversations because you never want to make a person feel like they are dying when they still have energy and zeal for life. At the same time, realism helps inform safety and the transition to the final stage of life. In most cases, an elderly loved one needs love and presence more than fanciful and dangerous delusions meant to buoy false hope.

When my friend wondered why I was not putting money away for retirement, he was equivalent to the cousin in the scenario. It was not his intention to make me feel bad. He was trying to help me plan and be financially stable and had no idea that it was absurd to think anything other than my best years were behind me. Like an elderly person slowly losing mobility, I was losing lung function, which affected my walk to work and walking up stairs. Those with chronic conditions who can feel their decline hastening and who are experiencing the deterioration of organs should not feel compelled to take on more responsibilities. Although it can be difficult to have these conversations and to make these decisions with the elderly, it isn't cruel. Rather, it honors people at the place they are in life. Honesty and discussion about what someone can do is the primary consideration.

During my work as a hospital chaplain, I listened to many elderly patients wrestle with the realization that they are declining. Sometimes patients bluntly say that they are ready to die. I do not mean they would harm themselves. Rather, they feel their affairs are in order and they have "lived a good life." Often their spouse has died, and their children are adults. They may have an impending sense of dread about a medical prognosis that may be painful or incurable. They know the end is near and have made some sense of peace with the transition to whatever they believe comes after this world. These encounters are powerful for any chaplain, but especially for someone living with a chronic illness. I have experienced these thoughts many times and had moments where I accepted my fate as unfair and uncontrollable. I felt a sense of empathy with these patients living in their equivalent of CF Time.

When speaking about these cases with one of the CPE educators at the Cleveland Clinic, Rabbi Jim Egolf offered that "the greatest lie we had ever been told is you have time." Most people think they have all the time they need to accomplish what they want in life because they live by the deliberate hour hand. Those who are dying in hospitals, or those who live with chronic conditions, may see this statement for what it is—a deception. Those with CF or other terminal illnesses who have been told by well-meaning folks that they "have time" to accomplish their goals understand the lie better than most people.

During my residency, I visited a man in his sixties on the surgical floor. He said he came into the hospital to have general tests and found out that morning he had cancer. Upon hearing this, my tone shifted, as I felt his sadness at the horrible and surprising turn of events. He may have picked up on this and strongly affirmed, "I'm not giving up. There is still a lot I want to do. I still have time." We explored how he wanted to "patch things up" with his son, as they had become estranged. He had the idea of writing him a letter, so if he died, his son would always have it. I encouraged him to write it and thought it might be helpful for their relationship. I made a note to follow up with him. A week later, he had been moved to the oncology floor. A few days later, I saw he was now in palliative care. Each time I came to see him, he seemed to be sleeping. The following week, he was moved to comfort measures only (CMO), a sign that active measures would no longer be taken to treat his underlying condition. The next day, he died. I never had a chance to speak with him again, to hear if he had reconciled with his son. After a mere two weeks since learning he had cancer, this man was dead. He thought he had time. The second hand was moving far quicker than either of us realized.

Carpe Diem

The diary entry at the start of chapter 1 recalls my attendance at the play *Our Town* in high school. I sat by myself toward the back of the auditorium and had no clue what the play was about before it started. During Act III, the Stage Manager (who represents an all-knowing God-like figure) takes Emily, the protagonist who has died, back to witness some impactful moments in her life. This process reveals something to Emily about the way human beings live. She breaks down crying and tells the Stage Manager, "I can't. I can't go on. It goes so fast. We don't have time to look at one another."[17] These lines struck me because I had begun to feel that CF Time was causing me to live my life in fast forward. I remember getting choked up when Emily watched her family and described her mother. I recall getting sad and thinking how much I would miss my own mother if I went back in time to look at happy moments, and how guilty I would feel if I died before my parents because I had CF.

Before returning to her grave, Emily asks the Stage Manager if "human beings ever realize life while they live it, every, every minute?" The Stage Manager pauses, and then replies, "No . . . the saints and poets maybe—they do some."[18] I recall sitting in my seat confused as the play came to an end. What would it mean to live as

---

17. Thornton Wilder, *Our Town: A Play in Three Acts* (Harper Perennial Modern Classics, reprinted 2003), Act III.
18. *Our Town*, Act III.

a "saint" or "poet" who sees the world differently? In that moment, I took it to mean being a good person who thinks deeply about life.

As I grew older, I gained a different understanding of what it means to be a saint when I encountered the works of Thomas Merton, a Trappist monk who wrote extensively on issues of justice, peace, and the environment. In *Seeds of Contemplation*, he writes, "For me, to be a saint means to be myself. Therefore, the problem of sanctity and salvation is the problem of finding out who I am and of discovering my true self."[19] As a high school student, and still today, it is difficult for me to accept my "true self" as a person with a chronic illness. Accepting that part of me is one way I work toward "realizing life" while I live it. It isn't easy, and I think it is important for someone with a chronic illness to come to accept the ways it can make life difficult. It is helpful when I allow myself the grace to grieve the challenges. I can't deny that I have CF, nor can I deny the way it has formed my understanding of time and what the future may hold. I need to give myself space and opportunity to be true to myself and live in a way that is authentic and genuine to who I am.

Merton explains that humans are unique in this struggle to be who they truly are. He writes, "A tree gives glory to God first of all by being a tree. . . . Trees and animals have no problem. God makes them what they are without consulting them, and they are perfectly satisfied."[20] There is a beautiful simplicity to realizing that trees and animals embrace their identity. If I had been able to be more like a tree, perhaps I would not have worked so hard to hide CF from other people. Perhaps I would have been able to focus more on living my life courageously and embracing CF, rather than hiding my true self. If *Our Town* is correct, perhaps saints and poets cherish life because they know how to be themselves, and they embrace their identity without apology or pretense.

---

19. Thomas Merton, "Things in their Identity," in *Seeds of Contemplation* (New Directions, 1949), 26.
20. Merton, "Things in their Identity," 24–26.

Emily's question of whether human beings "realize life while they live it" can also be unpacked.[21] She doesn't ask if people appreciate life. She asks if they "realize" life. Appreciating life may come in the form of expressing gratitude for opportunities, while realizing life is about possessing an awareness of each moment. For example, I can live in a state of gratitude, thankful for the way people have helped me or given me opportunities. Realizing life encompasses gratitude and so much more. To realize each moment means to see it in its fullness and to take hold of opportunities for growth. This is an important perspective because anyone can lose their health at any time. For some, it may mean living in some form of YOLO, as Reid described. For others, it might be living cautiously and preparing for death. Perhaps realizing life means rushing to accomplish things quickly because you know you don't have a long time to achieve your goals.

There are many ways that realizing life in CF Time might appear. Like Reid, Devin Broadbent, an aspiring actor, knew as a young person that CF could cut his life short. He was in the hospital often during his teenage years, and when he was sixteen he was told by his doctors, "Looking at your chart [lung function] you are probably on your way to transplant by the time you hit college. . . . Where do you see this going?" Devin was shocked. "As a sixteen-year-old, you hear this and think, 'Oh God.' And that conversation, knowing I had a shorter shelf life, changed all of my decisions." He worked as much as he could to save money and decided he would travel. He visited Australia and traveled as often as possible when he was not in the hospital. Devin reflected, "My idea was to try to see the world because it was the most reasonable thing I could do with the time I have left." For those who process CF Time like Devin, realizing life means experiencing the world before it is too late.

Ryne Beck, a strength and conditioning coach, took a different approach to his shortened life expectancy. He grew up in a disciplined household, which, along with having CF, has influenced how he sees the world. "I was told my life expectancy. . . . You

---

21. *Our Town*, Act III.

would think someone who is told their life expectancy would be living with the wind, wherever it takes you. I'm not like that." Ryne explained that he is a planner: "I have this finite time to lock in and cherish every moment I have with my family, but I need to be prepared for the medical bills, and my kids' school if I am not here, and the health insurance policy for my wife. Some people think it is morbid, but that is how I look at it." Ryne has tried to live a focused life within his means, both financially and in the way he has taken care of his body. He explained, "I know I probably won't live to retire, but if I start a Roth IRA and put it in a trust and then into my will, at least there is something for my wife and kids." For those who process CF Time like Ryne, realizing life means preparing his family for a time when he is no longer alive.

My perspective on realizing life may appear more like Ryne but it felt more like Devin. The knowledge of my death kept me moving at a fast pace. I set goals and worked to achieve them quickly. I studied hard in school and eventually achieved a PhD in systematic theology. My choice to stay in school wasn't about planning for my future; it was about living for the moment. I enjoyed school and had my education paid for through assistantships. I hoped to live long enough to become a teacher but knew that was not assured. At times, I prioritized the present over the future, especially in romantic relationships. Realizing life from my perspective meant focusing on what was happening in the moment. It helped me achieve my goals but was also sometimes harmful and sabotaging for my future.

Aside from the play, *Our Town*, I was also affected by the movie, *The Dead Poets Society*, which we watched in a high school theology class. In one scene, Mr. Keating, played by Robin Williams, takes his students to the hall to view photos of past students. He asks one of the students to read a selection of "To the Virgins, to Make Much of Time," by Robert Herrick. A student recites, "Gather ye rosebuds while ye may/ old-time is still a flying/ And this flower that smiles today/ tomorrow will be dying." Keating says that the Latin term for this sentiment is carpe diem. He elucidates, "We are food for worms, lads . . . each and every one of us in this room is one day going to stop breathing, turn cold, and die."[22] Keating tells them that the boys in the photos are not so different from them, as they all believed they were destined for great things. He asks, "Did they wait until it was too late to make from their lives one iota of what they were capable?"[23] He tells them that those in the photos are all fertilizing daffodils and they are whispering to the boys "carpe diem."

Many of my classmates seemed unmoved by this clip, at least based on their body language. Their heads were down, eyes closed, and some were talking to other students. I, however, was astonished. I remember feeling like I wanted to take on the world and run out of the room shouting "carpe diem!" It now makes sense that many of them were less moved because they were focusing on the hour hand of life, while I had begun to see the second hand. I had learned about Mr. Luedeke, had recently seen *Our Town*, and now Mr. Keating gave these realizations a new emotional outlet of excitement. I wanted to gather up the rosebuds while I could. I had no clue what that meant for me, but I knew it meant something. Following high school, I went on to college and graduate school, living out my realization of carpe diem by embracing my education. For Devin, it meant traveling the world before his health declined and made travel impossible. For Ryne, it meant he needed to ensure that his family was financially cared for after his death. We all seized the day in our own way because CF Time meant we had less time to make from our lives one iota of what we were capable of achieving.

James Richardson, a trainer, coach, and motivational speaker, offers a thoughtful way to synthesize realizing life and seizing the day. James struggled a lot with CF growing up, experiencing excruciating coughing spasms when he tried to sleep. "From the day we were born, life has been trying to take us out," James reflected. "Our minds can't wrap around the fact that I'm not going to be around for family and friends, and that takes a toll mentally and emotionally." For James, seizing the day means helping other

22. *Dead Poets Society*, directed by Peter Weir (Touchstone Pictures, 1989).
23. *Dead Poets Society.*

people to process what it means to have a chronic illness: "It has made me more empathetic and given me a strength that is a lot different than people who have never had to deal with something like that," he explained. "A lot of time we look at CF as a bad thing, which it is in a lot of aspects; but we also have to look at . . . what we get out of this on an emotional level. Being able to help others get through their pain," James has adapted his experience of living in CF Time to help other people dealing with illness and struggles. As a personal trainer, he helps people move from a victim mentality to realizing some of the strengths gained by overcoming struggle. He realizes life by challenging people to seize the day, even if the day is short. "We could be angry because of the cards we are dealt, but I have this illness and there is nothing I can do about it on a genetic level," he acknowledged. James empowers those who may not have a role model to reframe living with a terminal condition.

No one knows what the future holds. Those aware they are living in CF Time are pretty certain the future is a lot shorter. They have less time to accomplish their dreams and live with an awareness that decline can arrive at any moment. It may mean seizing the day because no other day is promised. It may encourage discipline, strength, and empathy, or cause feelings of exhaustion and disillusionment. Living in CF Time can be a gift that pushes achievement or a curse that creates emptiness and isolation. Those living in CF Time are often less gullible when they hear someone utter the greatest lie that has ever been told.

Chapter 2

The Illusion

I am so worried about tomorrow. For a week I have been preparing for the big day. I went to bed early each night and I went on two long runs. I drank a lot of water each day, too. Tomorrow I will wake up early, eat a big breakfast, and drink a bottle of water. My appointment is at 11:00 a.m., which is the same time as three months ago when I had a good test. I have to remember to sit up straight while I am in the waiting room because I think that makes a difference. There is no margin for error this time because I have that trip with my friends next month and I will be heartbroken if I can't go. I hate how CF causes me to let my friends down. I have to do things just like last time so I can get a good test score. Good night.

If CF Time means living with the conceptualization of a decreased life expectancy, CF Space encapsulates *how* a person manages life in CF Time. As with CF Time, CF Space is not exclusively a CF concept, nor should it be assumed every person with CF experiences CF Space. However, many people who spoke to me articulated similar experiences, especially when transitioning into adulthood. I suspect that many people with chronic illnesses will connect with some of these observations, stories, and insights about what it means to inhabit the "space" of decline and powerlessness.

Pushing the Boulder

Five years before I found myself making the decision concerning retirement contributions with the HR representative, I contemplated a different decision. I had taken a break from studying for my doctoral exams by reviewing my previous pulmonary function tests (PFTs). At this point, I had gone from being in the hospital for IV treatments approximately once a year to once every eight months. I saw that my breathing test scores were no longer regaining as much ground despite doing IV treatments for four weeks. A wave of hopelessness crept over me. Why am I studying for these exams when I continue to get sicker? How long will it be until I am doing IVs every six months or three months? If I was healthy enough to get a job, could I retain a job teaching with those restrictions? I stared out the window of the third floor and looked at a tree blowing in the fall wind in front of the house. The feelings of despair became tinged with anger and frustration. I do everything that I can and yet, I still get sicker.

At the age of seventeen, Rachael Russell saw her older sister Katherine undergo a lung transplant after being on the transplant list for only two weeks. Rachael also has CF. Her sister's rapid decline was not only emotionally difficult because someone she loved could die; it was also a harbinger of Rachael's future. She reflected, "It was a tough time. I remember feeling hopeless. It felt like, no matter how compliant [with treatments] we both were, or how hard we fought, or how positive we remained, this is where she ended up." Rachael's sentiment is an apt description of CF Space and describes how I felt looking at my PFTs. It is the realization that "doing everything" will never be "doing enough."

It seemed like I stared at the tree in my emotional malaise a long time, immobilized by the CF Space that Rachael described. Those feelings of futility eventually began to dissipate, giving way to an illumination. Maybe I could run? I had never been a runner. I kept myself healthy during my childhood by practicing a Korean martial art called *Soo Bahk Do*, which I did for twenty-two years. I am certain that this kept me well during my teenage and early adult years. But my inability to cough up the mucus from my lungs while in class made it only partially effective at airway clearance. Maybe running outside, which would allow me to expel mucus as I ran, would be more helpful? I was determined to try.

The next day, I approached a group of friends and asked if any of them would be willing to run with me. While most in the group demurred, Theresa offered to give it a try. She hedged my expectations by explaining, "I used to run and haven't for a while, so I am not fast at all." That evening, we ran together for the first time. It must have been a comical sight. I didn't know that "running shoes" existed and was bundled with multiple layers as if I was going for an evening stroll.

We jogged/walked for about twenty minutes and went just over a mile. Upon completing our run, I bent forward and crouched down in a yard. I felt the evening dew on my fingertips as I knelt in the grass. I began to cough and cough, expelling the mucus clogging up my small airways. I assured Theresa, who did not yet know the implications of having CF, that this was what I wanted. Although surprised at my coughing and a bit concerned, she stood next to me without making me feel like I was making her uncomfortable. I stood up a few minutes later, sweat pouring down my brow and my chest aching. Despite being exhausted and hurting, I began to smile. "I can do this," I thought. We set a time to run later in the week and my running career had begun. I believed I had taken some control back from the disease and could moderate my decline.

Brandon Miller, who lives in Idaho and works at Rockitecture Stoneworks as a stone engraver, was also inspired to run to maintain his health. "None of my doctors . . . pushed fitness much because back then it was, do your treatments and shelter your children. . . . It was . . . just keep them safe," Brandon recalled. His experience on his first run was reminiscent of my own. "It was brutal. Absolutely brutal. I stopped three or four times because I went out way too fast and was coughing so badly. And I was so out of breath. I was on my hands and knees just trying to get air into my lungs," he emotionally recollected about his first run with his girlfriend when he was twenty-three. But Brandon kept at it, knowing that keeping active was key to his longevity. Although he still coughed, over time, running became easier and he saw the positive benefits to an active lifestyle.

In 2012, Brandon ran his first half-marathon. Inspired by Emily Schaller, the founder of *Rock CF*, he chose to run in a race hosted by her foundation. "Emily was a big part of my fitness journey . . . in trying to give back to the CF community," Brandon explained. He hoped to inspire other people with CF to do more than they think is possible. "I want to show younger patients that you can do . . . as much as professional athletes. You just have to . . . put your mind to it and stick with it," he passionately stated. Brandon has continued to run races and defy the odds. It all began because he took a chance, with the woman who became his wife, at doing something that pushed him beyond what he thought he was physically able to do.

Coincidentally, I also ran the same half-marathon at Grosse Isle, in 2012. It was my first experience with *Rock CF*. I had reached a point in my life where I wanted to do something to help people with CF and I had begun to be a consistent runner. The race in 2012 was my fourth half-marathon, and I was able to clearly detect the way running aided my health. I continued to adhere to all my treatments. My lung deterioration slowed, and my IV hospitalizations hovered back to once a year, rather than declining to once every six months. I had achieved the goal I had set as I watched the wind blow through the trees. I was doing my best to keep CF at bay. I didn't allow myself to think long-term about how it might keep me alive. The goal was always to stave off IV treatments just a bit longer. I am grateful to the countless people who have run with me and helped me in this cause.

Battling CF from an early age, Emily Schaller, the founder of *Rock CF*, knew the power of physical fitness. The organization originally used music as a fundraiser for the *CF Foundation*. Emily held rock concerts and released CDs to raise money. Her growing awareness of the importance of physical health precipitated the transformation of her organization, from raising awareness through music to raising awareness through fitness. Emily reflected, "Once

I started running and biking in 2006, . . . the shift of the mission changed because I saw a direct benefit from exercise, and [it] improved my lung function." Emily credits exercise with keeping her well enough to benefit from the new technologies associated with CF care. Her organization has done a lot to impress upon people like Brandon and me the importance of exercise and lung health. *Rock CF* also makes it possible for people to run by collecting and distributing running shoes to those who need them. "We have donated 1700 pairs of shoes," she explained.

Each year from 2012 to 2018, I ran in the *Rock CF* half-marathon. By 2018, my half-marathon time was nearly three hours, and I knew my body was no longer able to go 13.1 miles.[24] Although running had kept me well for far longer than I expected that October day when I first jogged with Theresa, I knew it was not sustainable. I told myself I would walk the 5 km race the following year and continue to do so until I was no longer able to walk 3.1 miles. It was frustrating to see the debilitation of my lungs, knowing that no matter how much I trained or how many times I did my treatments, my body could no longer handle it. My airways were closing off. I was experiencing the decline of a person in the final stages of their life . . . and I was thirty-six years old. Running gave me some control in CF Space, but it was slipping away. Just as Rachael described, I had done everything I could to remain healthy, but it wasn't enough.

I previously used the fictional character Soran from *Star Trek: Generations* to emphasize the way time can be perceived as a predator. For some with a chronic condition, it is not time that is preying on them but the disease itself. At times, it seemed like CF was always taking something from me, piece by piece. I was watching parts of my life slowly slip away. It is difficult to maintain hope and a positive outlook when you are constantly buffeted by bad

---

24. As a reference for non-runners, my fastest time completing a half-marathon was 1 hour and 59 minutes. Adding roughly 10–15 minutes per year as my lungs declined was a constant depressive reminder that no matter how much I trained, I was losing lung health and capacity.

news and difficult prognoses. This was especially true in 2018, as I could only run in short spurts and then had to walk. Metaphorically, the disease was now running faster than me, despite my years of training. The disease doesn't take a break and doesn't need to stop for water.

A helpful image that shows how I felt during these years of decline is the story of Sisyphus, from Greek mythology. The gods of Mount Olympus punished Sisyphus and forced him to push a boulder up a hill. Each day he carried out his task, only to have the stone roll down the hill for him to roll it up again the next day. I can only imagine how the mythical character felt nearing the top of the summit, believing he had done the impossible, with a sense of accomplishment within. But then the rock descended back down the hill. It is easy for a rock to roll down a hill. It is hard to push it up. His punishment was to repeat this exercise again and again for eternity. The image of Sisyphus is commonly used to denote an impossible task.

I think of this image when I see months of work to stay healthy constantly being rolled back. This experience is common for people with chronic illnesses who have one instance of getting sick with a minor cold and then end up in the hospital for weeks, or for an elderly person who experiences a fall that precipitates other medical issues. I felt a sense of accomplishment when I had a good visit with my doctors or had a good run. All that work can quickly be undone with a bad visit or difficult run, where I can tell that my lungs are beginning to lose capacity. I wanted to tell myself that I was in control of the disease; in reality, the disease still held the final say. Like Sisyphus, each accomplishment was ultimately undone. The boulder going downhill is symbolic of my own inevitable descent.

One of the most frustrating indicators of decline is the PFT. The opening diary entry is a realistic reflection of how I felt prior to doing a PFT for much of my life. For a week, I would stress about this test, as it was often used as the barometer for my health. If the result dropped 5–7% from the previous test, it was deemed that my lungs were being restricted. My doctor would then offer a choice. I could try two or three weeks of oral antibiotics and return for another test or go straight to two to three weeks of IV antibiotics. The stakes were high. By my mid-twenties, the oral medications rarely made a difference, so I usually chose to go right to the IVs. But, if I had travel plans or an important event coming up, doing the two weeks of oral medication sometimes made it possible to wait longer for the aggressive treatments. The IVs often wiped out any running progress I had made because they were so debilitating. It was always a gut-wrenching choice, and there are risks. The IV medication is potent and can only be used so many times before your body begins to gain resistance. The drugs can also damage your liver, kidneys, and other organs. In order to kill the germs in your lungs, you risk killing other parts of your body. Those who suffer from other chronic conditions often have to do the same calculus. Is the risk and the pain of the treatment worth it when it may be worse than the disease?

In some ways, though, the worst part of the PFT was not the potential outcome of a bad test. It was the seeming unpredictability of the outcome. In the diary entry, I described behaviors I would do the week before doing the test and how I would sit in the waiting room. I often went into the test expecting a good score because I was running well, feeling good, and doing everything to take care of myself . . . only to hear my score was down 7% or more. It is a horrible feeling to know you are declining. It is even worse to hear that you are declining when you expect the opposite. When I would complain to my doctors, I was often told that the test can indicate small airway blockages before a person begins to feel sick and that it was important to do something sooner than later. The longer the wait, the more difficult to gain back that lost ground. My optimism that I had moved the boulder to the top was replaced by my shock of seeing it roll down, again and again.

To "beat" the test, I seized on random things—what I ate or drank, how much I ran the previous week, and any other advantage I could gain against the machine. For example, a few months after I began running, I had an FEV1 in the low 90s. It was one of the best scores I had ever had. I felt like I had cracked the code and that running, along with my daily treatments, was going to keep me healthy. Three months later, I did everything the same. I ran the same amount and went in with confidence. The test dropped nearly 20%. I was baffled, angry, and demoralized. A few days later, I began the IVs; meanwhile, the grief over realizing that I had not cracked the code remained long after the PICC line was withdrawn.

Erin McCaw is fifty-three. She described a similar experience with the PFT machine: "There would be times you would go in and you felt fine. And [they would say] we think you need to do some IVs. My sister and I, for the longest time, were convinced that if we had breath mints before, it helped us." Those who battle a seemingly unpredictable machine will do anything to gain an advantage, whether it be a hard run, breath mints, or extra sips of water. Like Rachel and me, Erin reasoned that doing the right things would produce a positive result. She explained, "We were . . . convinced that if you did everything precisely . . . you wouldn't get sick. . . . And then you show up . . . and it wouldn't matter how great your routine was. It was never quite good enough." This belief that doing everything perfectly meant not getting sick was a belief that originated with her parents and was reinforced during her CF clinic visits.

Erin and I also experienced blame from doctors when our PFT would decline. It was as though some doctors felt it was impossible to lose 7% in three months if someone was adhering to treatments. The machine can't be wrong; therefore, the human must be lying. This pressure can have all sorts of ramifications. Erin described how this experience in CF Space affected her mental health. She explained, "I think some clinics have gotten better at the mental health implications of telling a patient that they got sick because they haven't done something." In addition to the surprised disappointment of a low score is the shame of being made to feel like it is your fault. An unseen force didn't send the rock back down the mountain. It was because you didn't push it correctly.

One of the few times in my life I remember my parents crying is when I called them while driving home from a clinic checkup. I had left the house full of confidence that my score would be good, and I even assured my parents that the checkup would go well. When the score dropped 7–10% that day, I was devastated. The doctor said I would need to do IVs right away. I called my parents while driving home with tears in my eyes. My father answered the phone and said, "Clean bill of health? Tell us how good it went!" There was silence as I tried to mask my tears. "It wasn't good. I have to do IVs" is all I could muster without breaking down. I heard the pain in my parent's silence. "How can that be? You feel so good," my father said, his voice cracking with confusion and sadness. I heard my mom begin to cry. They wanted to support me but didn't know how. I vowed that day to never be the source of my parents' crying again, which meant hiding my decline from them, which is not healthy either. As someone in his mid-twenties with a chronic disease, I had inappropriately added the responsibility for my parents' emotional well-being to the list of heaviness that I carried leaving the clinic. The PFT machine won that day.

During my work as a hospital chaplain, I visited several people who expressed sadness and frustration over having a lack of control. One woman in her eighties who had fallen confided in me that she always takes care of herself and was so upset that this fall had happened and that it put her in the hospital. She did not want to be a burden to her family and could not accept that she had entered the age where falls can happen and can have deleterious effects on a person's health. When I raised these questions in my CPE internship class, my educator, Rev. Bob McGeeney, shared this powerful insight: "Control is an illusion." Bob, who has cancer, explained that the central issue for some patients is the lack of control over their lives, whether it is because of age or illness.

Bob's point is even more stark when people arrive in an ambulance and are awake and conversing with their loved ones, only to die a few hours later. In one of the most moving cases during my residency, I sat with a man whose wife came into the emergency room with chest pains. I walked him from the emergency room to the STEMI lab[25] where they would be working on her heart. As we made the long walk, he conversed with me about his day,

25. The STEMI (ST-segment elevation myocardial infarction) lab is where a patient would be sent if experiencing heart attack symptoms.

53

demonstrating very little anxiety in his voice. He had just spoken to his wife when she got out of the ambulance, and he appeared confident that she would be okay. While we waited together for the doctors to give him more information, he described where he and his wife had gone to dinner the previous night. Unbeknownst to either of us, doctors were performing CPR, two doors away. They were not able to resuscitate her. I felt this case powerfully in my heart because it reminded me how fragile life can be. One minute the woman was having chest pain, and a few hours later she was gone. This man's life changed forever. He had no idea when he woke up that morning that it would be the last time he would wake up beside the woman he had loved for many years.

The more I reflected on the fallacy of control, the more I realized Bob was right. Seeing patients day after day who are declining and/or dying wakes one up to the reality of how little control humans have over their lives, regardless of how much money or power one has or how healthy someone is in their youth. Disease and debilitation can strike anyone. As Erin reflected, "I think we all have this illusion of control . . . which can . . . end up making you feel like you are constantly failing." I am not saying that we should not take care of ourselves and try to remain healthy. I am also not insinuating that having more money or access to modern healthcare doesn't make a difference in longevity. It certainly does, and that is why increased access to modern medicine is an important social justice goal. My point is that we can keep a disease or condition at bay. We can live our lives in the healthiest way possible. But that never makes us impervious to mortality. Eventually, the boulder will roll downhill. Ultimate control over our physical health is an illusion.

What Is Warrior Mentality?

When I was training in the martial art *Soo Bahk Do*, I had many excellent instructors who taught me self-awareness just as much as self-defense. One of my instructors was Dr. John Johnson. He holds a PhD, is a certified 8th degree Midnight Blue Belt,[26] a master instructor in *Soo Bahk Do*, and lives with spina bifida.[27] One day he asked me to work out with him to prepare for a national demonstration. Following our workout, he told me, "Jimmy, most people do not know what it is like to face battle. You and I face battle every day." I was nineteen and only beginning to know the conflict that awaited me, but I saw what he faced. He was one of the most proficient and intimidating martial artists in our organization. Dr. Johnson had adapted his training throughout his life so that his perceived weakness could be harnessed as a strength.

Dr. Johnson's reference to the daily battle refers to a conflict in the mind between the doubts of others and belief in oneself to achieve. Other people may think a person with spina bifida or cystic fibrosis is incapable of achieving things. Having confidence, supported by competence and effective performance, is a key to winning this battle. Belief comes first, followed by action. Dr. Johnson explained to me years later, "Belief and stereotypes about what you or someone else thinks you can't do become mere illusion in the face of direct performance of what 'can't' be done." I thought of his statement about facing battle often while running. Amidst the constant coughing and pounding of my chest, I was doing something people thought a person with CF couldn't do. These beliefs became an illusion with every step I took in my running shoes.

Within the CF community, one popular way to refer to those with CF is cystic fibrosis "warrior." This label seeks to exemplify that living with CF is a constant battle for the individual, as well as one's friends and family. There are also limitations to this paradigm. While it is fair to say a person is battling the disease, what if a person no longer wants to fight? Do they lose the label in disgrace? Also, how do we define "victory" and "loss" using warrior language?

---

26. A Midnight Blue Belt in *Soo Bahk Do* is equivalent to a Black Belt in other styles.
27. Spina bifida is a type of neural tube defect (NTD) that occurs when a baby's neural tube fails to develop or close properly prior to birth. The condition has a range of severity.

Andy Lipman has a special connection to the CF warrior image. A fifty-year-old husband and father of two, he compiled stories into a book entitled, *The CF Warrior Project*. These vignettes demonstrate different perspectives on living with CF. The decision to use warrior in the name comes from the way Andy sees the CF battle. He explained, "We have to deal with so much—not just the physical side, but the emotional side too. You get knocked down so many times, but you have to get back up. To me, that is a warrior." Andy recently published a second volume, expanding the label of those who are called CF warriors: "I used to think the only qualification was you had to have CF, and I said, maybe you don't." While writing the second book, he thought about his mother who was born in a displaced persons' camp in Germany following the Holocaust and whose love supported him growing up. Andy explained, "I thought about her perspective as a CF mom. So, I told her story and several CF mom stories." Andy's drive to raise funds for CF research also comes from his sister, who died, after a few weeks of life, from CF complications. To honor her, he created the nonprofit *Wish for Wendy Foundation Inc.*, which has raised over $4 million for the *CF Foundation*. As Andy continues the warrior's battle, he carries the memories of his mother and his sister, whose life was taken by CF before she ever met him.

One of the members of the CF community who exemplifies warrior mentality is Jerry Cahill. Jerry, who is in his late sixties, has survived three transplants. In 2012, he had a lung transplant, followed by a liver and kidney transplant in 2021. He had five dry runs (coming to the hospital for the transplant only to discover the organ is not suitable) and was able to receive lungs on the sixth attempt. Ten years later, he began to have liver issues. Jerry explained, "The . . . heart and the lungs work together. The liver and the kidneys work together. They . . . told me that at some point I was going to need a liver transplant." His kidneys also began to get worse. In July 2021, he was in the hospital for dialysis, and they told him he wasn't going to be able to go home. "They gave me a 20% chance of getting through the surgery," he explained.

After sixteen and a half hours, he pulled through. Such a battle epitomizes warrior mentality.

Like Emily, Brandon, and me, Jerry credits a strong workout routine in his younger years for making him healthy enough to have these transplants. "I think exercise is a great form of therapy, both mentally and physically," Jerry explained. His commitment to exercise and healthy living led him to work with the *Boomer Esiason Foundation*, which raises money and awareness for the CF community. Jerry explained, "Boomer allowed me to bring in exercise, and I created Team Boomer, which is the athletic leg of the foundation. Our goal is to support the CF community and advocate for them to live fuller and better lives." Jerry continues to do speaking engagements, fundraisers, and other activities to support the foundation. Like many people with CF, Jerry's work has touched countless lives, and his life is a powerful example of the warrior mentality that Andy described. When you get knocked down, it is possible to get back up and to keep fighting. When you see the boulder roll down the hill, it may call on something within you to push it back up the hill. That is the warrior mentality.

While the warrior image can be helpful, it is also important to acknowledge its limitations. Debra Mattson, who is fifty-three and lives in Canada, agrees. She cautions that "CF warrior" needs to be explained or it could create unrealistic expectations. Debra explained, "I think you have to leave room for people that, just because they are dying, doesn't mean they weren't fighting, and they are allowed to stop fighting." She continued, "It makes me cringe when we use that word and just let it go [without explaining it]." Her reaction partly comes from her perspective of CF as a child. She recalled, "When I was growing up, there was a fundraising poster on my wall that said, 'Julie is twelve years old. She has just reached middle age.'" Growing up knowing that she had a shortened life expectancy impressed upon her that life would be a battle. Like the warrior label, it can have harmful effects, creating an environment where one thinks that continuing to battle is the only answer. There may come a time when someone reaches the end, and any other measures should not be imposed upon someone who has fought the final battle. Everyone dies eventually.

I have thought of the importance of this distinction when patients in the hospital told me, "Chaplain, I am ready to die." They were usually elderly people with debilitating conditions who had reached a point where they were ready to stop fighting against the inevitable. While this can be hard to hear, it should not be viewed, in these cases of an elderly person with a serious condition, as "giving up." There needs to be a balance between the warrior mentality of continuing the fight, and the acknowledgment that it is time to rest. Both require courage. There is not a cookie-cutter definition of the difference. It is an awareness, a feeling, and a willingness to meet the other person where they are. Sometimes it means encouraging them to keep fighting, while at other times it means creating space so they do not feel guilty letting go.

During my residency, I came to the bedside of an elderly man who had died. His daughter was sitting by his bedside holding back tears. She explained that her father always told her how important she was to him and that he loved seeing her. The previous night, his health had begun to decline more than expected, from heart failure complications. He was still alive and aware of her presence when she arrived that morning for her daily visit. He died a few minutes later. I reflected with her that he may have fought as hard as possible to stay alive so she could see him one last time. Their bond appeared as meaningful to him as it was to her. This man was no less a warrior at his death than at any other time during his battle with heart disease. Realizing that the end has come and accepting death can be even more heroic than fighting for life.

In some visits, it became apparent that the patient and family member were approaching the patient's illness differently. In one case, I sat at the bedside of a man in his late eighties who had been a veteran and had traveled the world. He reflected fondly about his experiences, as his wife, who appeared in much better health, sat next to me. Any time the man would return to the present, he would sound less optimistic and become emotional. "I just don't know," he would share sadly, shaking his head. His wife, sensing this tone, would immediately jump into the conversation and say, "It will be fine. We will get through this." The man would grow silent. It appeared to me that she was in denial about his condition. I returned to see him the next morning, before she arrived, to create a space for him to share without pressure. He broke down in tears and acknowledged that he thought he might be at the end of his life and that he was ready to die, except he did not want to leave his wife. I encouraged him to have these hard conversations with her so that she understood that he was ready to stop fighting.

A patient becoming CMO can also be an example of "ceasing" to fight. As a chaplain, I had discussions with family members where they offered that it was the patient's wishes to not be in a certain condition, such as dependent on food, hydration, or a respirator. Sometimes people question, "I know this is what he wanted, but it is still very hard. Are we doing the right thing?" This uncertainty sometimes comes from believing that one must morally do everything to live. Most philosophical and religious traditions, however, leave space for the morality of "letting die" when it is deemed that all measures have been taken and that extending life is painful and burdensome.

The importance of defining warrior mentality applies to all chronic health conditions. If a warrior is a person who lives with burdens that others do not, I think it is a meaningful distinction. For example, a person who is living with a slowly debilitating illness will be fighting to do things one day that were easier the days and weeks before. Basic daily activities can take courage, strength, and fortitude. This person is displaying warrior mentality. However, if the description is used to describe what a person *should* do in the future, it can be problematic and even detrimental. This is evident in the case of the man whose wife continued to pelt him with optimistic platitudes. An ill person who thinks they *should* keep fighting their disease, lest they "fail," can have a burden put upon them that becomes prescriptive, rather than descriptive. The warrior label isn't a merit badge for suffering longer and harder than anyone else; it is commendation for living with a debilitating circumstance that no one else will ever understand.

Paul Fugelsang, a psychotherapist who specializes in treating anxiety, depression, and trauma, offers a great metaphor to help understand CF Space. Paul asks people to imagine carrying daily burdens like carrying a bag of rocks. Each encounter with a person can take a rock away (make their day lighter) or add a rock to their bag (make their day more difficult). For example, stopping to ask how someone is doing or helping someone carry something might remove a small rock. Conversely, making fun of someone, belittling them, and singling them out could add a rock to their bag. He challenges people to do what they can to remove rocks instead of adding them.[28]

I find Paul's metaphor especially applicable to the chronic illness community. As Andy described, we carry around heavy "bags" more often than not. Medications, doctor appointments, mental health, physical health, and the way our conditions impact those we love are all ways our bags are routinely heavy. It is as though CF Space is a large, ever-present rock. But there are ways to chip away at this boulder and each speck makes the bag lighter. Those with the heaviest bags are most aware of when something has been removed, and in many cases, they are the most grateful. In this analogy, perhaps what Sisyphus most needs is not someone to help push the rock up the hill, but someone to chip away at it, to make it lighter. He still has to push the rock. No one can push it for him. One can't take the pain away from those we love who have a chronic illness but making the rock a bit lighter could mean all the difference in the world. Chipping away at the size of the rock isn't an illusion of controlling it, but rather, accepting it and fighting to live. A slightly lighter rock is one way to fight a bit longer in CF Space.

---

28. James Menkhaus, *Immersion: A Pilgrimage into Service* (New City Press, 2022), 127–129.

Chapter 3

The Long Loneliness

I hate going to dinner in the dining hall. I always try to go at 4:25 so I can be done by 5:00, but tonight I had to go at 6:00 because of that meeting. It was like everyone was looking at me. I sat on the far side hoping no one could tell I was eating alone. I sat one of my books in front of me so it looked like I was studying and that is why I was eating alone. I wonder what people would think if they knew I didn't have any friends here. I ate as fast as I could. I think I was out by 6:15. As I left, I saw everyone cracking jokes and laughing with their friend groups. I feel like they are laughing at me. I wish I didn't always have to eat alone. At least the rest of the week I can go when the dining hall opens so no one will see me. I feel like the only person who eats alone. Good night.

Along with CF Time and CF Space, there is also CF World, which I will use to refer to the way of living with a chronic illness that can include long periods of isolation and despair as one grows into the realization of being different from everyone else. These differences can bring ridicule from peers, self-doubt and shame, or the feeling that you will never be in a romantic relationship. Not everyone with a chronic condition will be able to relate to each example but I suspect many will understand some of the challenges with building relationships for people deemed by society as "different." For some with a chronic condition, community is a crucial aspect to being able to stay well, and yet, it can be one of the most difficult components of living each day. Loneliness is even more unpalatable when you feel no one will ever understand the lens through which you encounter the world.

Marooned on an Island

I grew up in a small exurb in Cincinnati, Ohio called Indian Ridge. The Sanzone, Miller, and Mattingly families all had children near my age. It was a ten-minute drive to the nearest grocery, and we were isolated on "the hill," away from much of the world. I don't remember the time when each of these friends discovered I had CF. It likely filtered down from my parents to their parents to their children. I was the child who didn't get to do sleepovers with these friends, nor could I play outside when it got cold. Only rarely was I permitted to join a snowball fight, and I never went sledding. Beyond that, these childhood relationships were not encumbered greatly by my condition. The hill was a safe space for me to be myself and these friends never made me feel different.

Outside of the safe confines of Indian Ridge, however, I never spoke about having a medical condition. I had very few friends outside of this community. I did my best to hide visits to the school nurse after each meal so as not to appear "different." One minor difference can make you the object of ridicule of your classmates. In grade school, I was absent more than most kids due to common illnesses. In high school, coughing became a new part of my CF experience. It is likely I didn't do as good of a job hiding my illness as I thought, but I tried my best. I saw it as my private life, my weakness, that no one needed to know. I didn't want to be different from everyone else. The thought never occurred to me that other children might be hiding their own issues that made them feel the same way.

Maddie Core, who recently graduated from college, doesn't think that having CF made her much different from other children most of the time either. She recalled, "Sometimes my friends, when I was young, would ring the doorbell and would want to go outside

and play, and I couldn't because I hadn't done my treatments yet."
She also remembers being in kindergarten with a PICC line. "You
know kindergarteners," she reflected smiling. "They don't care,
they will be like, 'What is that in your arm?'" One experience she
remembers caused her to be "really embarrassed about having CF."
She reflected on a grade school trip to Washington, DC: "There
was a teacher who had all the meds and so I would try to go to her
in secret because I didn't want anyone to know I had CF." Many
children with CF take medication with meals, and wanting to hide
that is a common reaction. Despite these moments, Maddie expressed
that having CF was not a huge barrier to overcome as a child.

While growing up in New Zealand, Nick Laing had a different
CF childhood experience. "I got bullied quite a bit as a kid," he
confided. Because of his additional nutritional needs, he ate lunch
with the school staff. This caused him to be a target of ridicule by
other children because they knew he was different in some way.
Having CF also caused Nick to miss school a lot. By his twelfth
year, he had to spend six months being homeschooled because he
was too sick to attend school with everyone else. Being chronically
ill and different from others, especially as a child, can make school
and other social activities difficult experiences of isolation. Nick's
experience of missing core memories in school and constantly
fighting illnesses is a common occurrence in the chronic illness
community.

High school is when my lungs began to show typical signs of
CF through a constant cough. My classmates would often refer to
it as "chronic bronchitis" and would ask "Will you ever get better?" I was too afraid to be vulnerable and truthful. I would just
tell them I wasn't getting well, and I wasn't sure if I ever would.
Mr. Luedeke's decline loomed in my mind. I thought that perhaps
my disease was even worse than his and I wouldn't make it to my
twenties without a lung transplant. During my junior year of high
school, I wondered if I would be healthy enough to attend college.

Zack Swanborn, who is currently twenty-four, explained another
hurdle to having CF during high school—complying with treatments. Unlike me, whose early high school time pre-dated the vest

and nebulizers, Zack wrestled with balancing time with friends and his daily treatment regimen. "You are in eighth grade, ninth grade, and you want to be like all the other kids, and you just don't want to do it. You want to stay out late and have fun," he confided. If the vest had been available to me, I would have wrestled with the same questions. Having to leave a friend's house to do medical treatments isn't something any child wants to do. Zack went on to explain, "I think that noncompliance . . . contributed to popping the cork. . . . I broke the seal on the decline in my lung function." It can be hard for a seemingly healthy child to understand the importance of daily treatments. While it is a challenge for adults to adhere to strict treatments amidst the busyness of life, teenagers may have even more things that they would rather be doing.

Attending college with a chronic illness presents unique challenges. College can be a very difficult time for students, especially those who are introverted and different in some perceived way. I chose to leave Cincinnati to attend John Carroll University (JCU) in Cleveland, Ohio. I distinctly remember my CF doctor and parents being doubtful whether I would make it and expecting me to return home before the end of the first year. I was moving to a colder climate and was taking my new vest, inhalers, and medications. Ironically, it was not my health, nor my studies that I found the most challenging. It was navigating social relationships while trying to hide a chronic disease from everyone else in the college dorm.

Before choosing to attend JCU, my parents coordinated with the housing department to make sure I could have a single room with a bathroom. There were only a few such rooms on campus. It was a nonnegotiable for me to be able to clean my inhalers and to not have a random roommate. Donna Byrnes, Director of Residence Life, assured me she could make it possible. For the next four years, when the housing selection process began, Donna always helped me select a single room with a bathroom. She was one of the unsung heroes of my college experience. Without her, I would not have been able to attend JCU.

However, this accommodation also made it difficult for me to make friends. It was a double-edged sword. I always kept my door closed because I did not want people to see my medical equipment and inhalers. When people saw that I had a single, it always led to questions: Why does this guy get a bathroom? After the first weekend, I began to keep my door closed all the time. I worried that people passing by could hear me coughing or doing my treatments. I tried to mask the sound of my treatments by doing them when the dorm was the loudest. In my first year of college, only one person visited my room (to pick up a book) and I never went into someone else's room.

Talia Cestone, from Pennsylvania, also moved away from home to attend college. She was lucky to get an understanding roommate. "She was very supportive . . . and helped me figure out doing treatments around practice. It became part of her mission," Talia reflected. She had a close group of friends who knew [about her situation] but was slow to tell others. Talia reflected on an evening when she and her friends were preparing to go out. "I had [my treatments] going and there were three friends over," she explained. There was a knock on her door, and she immediately went into protective mode. "No one can know about this; no one can see any of this," she reacted. One of her friends told the girl at the door that they were vacuuming and would be out in a moment. "[The girl] rolled with it, and I appreciated that," reflected Talia. Her story affirms the importance of having a few trusted friends while being circumspect in choosing who to tell about one's condition.

The fear of coughing in class was a constant concern for both Talia and me during college. "I hated the way it sounded. . . . The more I tried to stifle it in class, or for a prolonged period, it's like it's brewing [in my lungs]," she explained. One cough could trigger a chain reaction or coughing fit that would disturb a class. When Talia coughed extensively, she would be asked the dreaded question, "Do you smoke?" Like Talia, I constantly got that question from people. "You should cut back a pack per day, buddy. Those things will kill ya," I heard more times than I can count a stranger offering "helpful" advice. I would politely respond, "Oh, I know," or "Don't worry, I don't smoke," as the person walked away chuckling.

"I hated it when people thought that [I smoked]," reflected Talia, "I was already so self-conscious of it."

The coughing bouts that Talia describes had become an issue for me as well. Constant coughing contributed to the alienation I felt from my peers. Unfortunately, there are many reasons people are ostracized in society. Differences in religion, politics, skin color, sexual orientation, and body image are prevalent reasons for exclusion. Sometimes, these barriers are created out of fear for one's own safety. Even though my time in college was well before COVID-19, a chronic cough communicates disease of some sort. Imagine that you are preparing to introduce yourself to a new classmate or colleague at work. As you approach, they begin to cough repeatedly and you can tell they need to expel mucus from their lungs, but because they are in public, they keep it contained in their mouth. Are you still as likely to go over and introduce yourself? Even a well-intentioned person is less likely to risk their health to reach out to a sick stranger.

I do not want to insinuate that people with CF have no friends. Rather, I want to raise the issue that those with chronic illnesses, especially those conditions that manifest in ways that seem to pose a health threat to others, face unique challenges when trying to form friendships. I think the image of an island describes how I felt at different points in my life. In literature, an island often denotes a closed community where things happen removed from society. People are marooned on islands, such as in *Robinson Caruso* or *Lord of the Flies*. One of my favorite series, *Lost*, uses the island as a place of mystery following an airplane crash. The chronic illness island can be a lonely place that isolates people from others.

The diary entry that began this chapter was repeated nearly every evening, as I ate most meals alone during the first two years of my collegiate experience. By my junior year, I found a group of friends who accepted me for who I was, but two years on the island formed the way I understood and experienced loneliness. As a teacher, I tell students to look for classmates who eat alone every day and invite them to join their table. They may say no, which is their right. Or, they may just be waiting for someone to truly see them, rather than the way society sees them, as an outcast who is different from others. I try to encourage others to seek out those who appear marginalized and lonely, despite sitting in a huge crowd. It takes a brave person to traverse the seas and risk illness to unlock the enigma of another person's loneliness.

Dorothy Day, the Catholic activist and founder of the Catholic Worker Movement, wrote an autobiography that she entitled *The Long Loneliness*. In one of the most quoted lines from her book, she explains, "We have all known the long loneliness and we have found the answer is love and that love is community."[29] I have always found this quote to be a beautiful articulation of the pain of isolation balanced with the healing balm of community. It is also inclusive, as Day asserts that we *all* know an aspect of what it means to be lonely. Historically, Day and the Catholic Worker Movement sought out those who were outcasts in society because of their socio-economic status or because they were experiencing homelessness. Day's creation of the Catholic Worker community for those "outcasts" became a way of helping them to find purpose and a supportive community.

Navigating the disclosure of a chronic illness and trying to form friends does not end when entering adulthood. Every time I meet new people, I am faced with the question of health transparency. How honest should I be about my debilitating health? In 2019, I began a new job and quickly became friends with Martha. I wanted her to know about my health condition in case I began to decline. I invited her to dinner, where I could reveal that aspect of myself that I felt needed to be hidden. It was very difficult for me to tell her, but I eventually worked it into the conversation. It wasn't that I was afraid of her judgment; I just did not want her to treat me differently. I never talked about having CF in my classroom because I didn't want to be "the teacher with CF," nor did I want to be known that way among my colleagues. Martha accepted my vulnerability graciously. She then reciprocated and explained that she identified as a member of the LGBTQ+ community, something that was also

---

29. Dorothy Day, *The Long Loneliness* (HarperCollins, 1952), 286.

not widely known. As I left dinner, I felt I had gained a friend who trusted me with part of herself and someone that I could be honest and vulnerable with as well. Sharing my story with Martha was difficult for me, but our friendship continues to remind me about the transformative potential of authenticity, that there are other good people who welcome friendship, and it may take vulnerability to find them. In rare instances, people visit the island. Usually, those who also feel the unjust pressure from society to hide aspects of their true selves enjoy the visit the most.

Chronic illness can also complicate romantic relationships. If a person is living on CF Time, how might that change the search for a romantic partner? If a person is living in CF Space and fighting each day to survive, how does that impact the mutual care that a couple promises to give to each other? The CF World of romantic relationships is fraught with difficult questions. As my mentor, Fr. Howard Gray, SJ, once told me, "Jimmy, relationships are difficult because you are dealing with the freedom of another person." This is especially true when you have a chronic illness. Taking care of a partner who becomes sick will likely impinge upon the freedom of the caregiver, as their needs and aspirations may take a back seat to the needs of the ill or aging loved one. When a person does not realize the ramifications of commitment, relationships can fall apart. This is true in every relationship but they may fall apart sooner when a chronic illness is involved. However, there are a variety of ways a person with a chronic disease can approach these types of relationships.

Bonnie-Rose Wise is currently a college student studying equine science. When she was younger, dating with CF wasn't a huge deal, but as she gets older, she sees that dating with a chronic illness is complex. "It is definitely changing a lot. I'll bring it [CF] up and they [potential date] will do a Google search and the first thing that comes up is forty years [life expectancy]," she expressed. Even if that may not be true for her because she feels relatively healthy, that is a difficult way to begin a relationship. "How do you put that on somebody else?" she reflected. "We have grown up with CF, and we are used to it. There is no other way of life. How do you take this disease and put it on somebody else and be like, are you ok with this?" Bonnie-Rose acknowledged that CF could get really bad, especially toward the end of someone's life. While a person with CF may be aware of the potential ramifications of old age, a person with CF who is in a relationship must make sure that their partner understands the ramifications as well; a partner of a person with CF could become a caretaker much earlier in life. Not everyone is willing to do this.

For much of my life, I wrestled with the same questions as Bonnie-Rose. I remember in high school saying to a girl I had a crush on, "I don't think we should date. I don't know how long I have to live, and I am just going to get sick." I was definitely looking ahead with optimism that we would end up getting married from a high school date! I really liked this girl, so I did not want her to fall in love with me because she would be sad when I died. On one hand, I very much desired to be in a relationship, as many people do during their teenage years. On the other hand, CF Time had colored the lens through which I viewed future possibilities, and relationships were another casualty of my approach. I am not saying I was right or wrong, I am simply pointing out the way I saw the possibility for a loving, long-term relationship. As Bonnie-Rose said, how could I place those expectations onto someone else?

Marina Finnell, who recently started law school, described some of the difficulties with dating with CF. "For me, CF was more challenging with relationships and trying to figure out how to have a partner in life," she explained. Marina has had a number of long-term relationships, but they eventually ended. "CF is a big deal, and at one point your partner is going to have to be a caregiver in a big way," she reflected. Marina feels CF frightened some people from a long-term commitment. "There are some people I've dated for a year or two and at the end of the day, they were not there during hospital stays or couldn't keep up with the intricacies of my doctor's appointments and IV regimen," she reminisced. Being with someone, but then feeling like you are being abandoned during your time of need, can be very detrimental to your belief in your self-worth.

When dating, I often wondered what is the best time to admit I have a chronic disease. There is some wisdom in leading with it. That is Marina's approach: "It is a first date thing [for me]. I say, here is what is going on, please don't waste my time." I can also see the perspective that it is better to wait a few dates. However, the longer you wait, the more you risk making the other person feel like you are withholding something important, especially if you have been coughing and they asked if you are sick, and you responded with obfuscation. It doesn't seem right to not ground a date in honesty, but what time is the right time? There is no established playbook for dating while you are dying.

Although much of my life I have taken an approach toward relationships that emphasized their temporary status, I was engaged when I was in my mid-twenties. My health had plateaued slightly, and I figured I had a few years with someone who I loved. We had discussions about what it would mean for me to not be able to have biological children because of CF.[30] We also discussed how she would handle being a young widow if I got sick and died, which seemed inevitable. Although I think we both did our best to be honest with each other, we were discussing things that were beyond our experience. I suspect that we rushed things because of the countdown of CF Time. Ultimately, we broke off the engagement.

At the time, I viewed that as my only chance at getting married, since I was still young enough to have a few healthy years with someone. Although I have dated since that time, I have always been upfront with people that I did not see the relationship leading to marriage. Most of the time, the relationship became short-lived when she began to understand that my approach was not typical of someone my age. Some people date for fun, while others look for someone they want to spend the rest of their life with. I would never allow myself to desire a long-term relationship knowing each healthy tomorrow could be my last.

---

30. Most men with CF are commonly born without a vas deferens, thus sperm are unable to travel to the semen. Women can also experience fertility issues.

Eliza Callard, a poet who lives in Philadelphia, thought as I did, in her twenties, until she fell in love with Emily. "I started having panic attacks. I am going to put this person through this terrible, terrible ordeal," she recalled. She also did not want CF to take away something that so many humans value—falling in love. "It felt right. This is part of being a human," Eliza affirmed. When they got together, Eliza was not sure how long she would be healthy. "We said to each other, if we can just have five years together, it will be amazing," she reflected. Now, Eliza and Emily have been together twenty-five years. They took a chance knowing that CF Time would play a predominant role in their lives, and they are thankful they took the risk. "I just decided I had met this incredible woman, and she was okay with it," Eliza reflected with a smile. Sometimes the island of loneliness can become an island of love shared with another person.

CF Time and CF Space can play a role in the criteria for a partner. If a person grows up expecting to be sick and to slowly deteriorate, finding a partner who can offer supportive care becomes an overriding criterion. Ryann McCoy, who lives in Texas, explained, "I worried about finding someone who would take care of me when I am sick. That was always my big concern." She acknowledges that this may not have been the best approach to finding a partner. "My mom put it in my head when I was little, 'You're not going to be able to do these things, and people aren't going to want to deal with your CF.'" She also acknowledged that she dated a few guys who read about CF and then "got creeped out," much as Marina described. Ryann has now reached a point where she knows what she is looking for, and that is more helpful for her and for those she will date in the future. "I think before I was looking for the wrong reasons, and now I actually want a partner and not a caregiver," she concluded.

Letting someone set foot on the island takes courage. One evening during my chaplain residency, I was asked to visit a patient late in the evening in the intensive care unit. He was quite ill and was suffering from a host of medical conditions. We spoke for a long time about his life. He described how a vehicle accident changed his life for the worst and that since then, he had been dealing with physical discomfort. At the end of his story, I asked if any family had visited him in the hospital. He paused and labored to breathe. "No," he replied. "Most of them are dead and my brother isn't well enough to travel."

I realized that this man was facing these challenges alone. I saw he was on an island experiencing the long loneliness. His illness, which caused him to have bouts of frustration with nurses, served to isolate him even more. When I had to leave to answer a page, I thanked him for sharing with me. He replied, "You have good bedside manner. . . . Thank you for listening." Perhaps it was the empathy I felt at his loneliness that kept me sitting with him for as long as I did. One might say I experienced projection, the term used in CPE when we see our story in the story of the patient. Sometimes it can be a "hook" that negatively influences your patient interaction, but if it is balanced correctly, it can also be a source of empathy. I do not claim to have a clue about "what he was going through," but I do know that in my life I have felt lonely and isolated. We shared a common human experience. We shared the similar feeling of being marooned on an island of isolation.

Six Feet Apart

Most health conditions have an aspect of shared solidarity in undergoing a health challenge. When I began training to be a hospital chaplain in the summer of 2023, I realized that COVID patients are not always isolated from each other. On one hand, this seemed odd because I had been formed by the previous three years of hearing about COVID-19 "isolation." However, COVID-19 patients cannot infect each other with COVID. One might be very sick, while another is less so, but the disease communicability is no longer a danger. It makes sense to conserve resources, and sharing a room may help the patient to know they are not isolated from everyone. Whether dying or recovering, they do not have to share those moments alone. Similarly, cancer patients can sit together in the same space while receiving chemotherapy, just as dialysis patients can be in the same space while undergoing treatment. I am not contending people immediately understand what someone else is experiencing. Rather, I point out that at minimum a person can see they are not physically isolated by their condition, and perhaps this helps them during treatment and potential recovery.

The possibility for shared community among those with CF, however, is very different than nearly every other medical condition. This is because those with CF must isolate themselves from all other people with CF at all times. This curious abnormality among shared underlying health conditions exists because of the possibility for cross contamination of bacteria. A person with CF is immediately put in isolation when at a CF clinic. At CF fundraisers or conferences, there is a strict attendance policy that only one person with CF may be admitted. Could you imagine a fundraiser for another medical condition where everyone can come, except those who have that condition?

If those with CF are momentarily in proximity, the official guidelines from the *CF Foundation* are to remain six feet apart. Long before "six feet apart" was the tagline for COVID safety, the CF World was attempting to navigate this policy among each other. Just as it left many people feeling disconnected during the pandemic, it continues to leave the CF community feeling detached. Bonnie-Rose articulated the difficulty with this policy: "So, no one really knows what you are going through. And then you're taught, stay six feet apart. . . . The only people who understand can't talk to you." Bonnie-Rose continued, "People with other diseases . . . they'd have support groups, and they can go sit in a circle and talk about it." Those with CF can't do this.

Talia also reflected on this difficult aspect of having CF. "So isolated. So isolated. That, I think, is the missing piece [of having CF]. Truly, no one understands," she said, raising her voice. The emotional toll became more apparent as she shared a story of a brief encounter, in the waiting room at her clinic, with another person who had CF:. "One day, before COVID, there was a girl [with CF] in the waiting room. We both were there for appointments and had masks on. She was very forward and sat next to me, and I should have gotten up, but I didn't. . . . It was a very brief conversation, but I wanted to suck in as much information as I could get from her." It was clear how this short encounter impacted Talia, as she told the story with her voice becoming louder and more excited. I suspect it was like meeting someone you didn't know existed, but also the first time talking to someone who may really understand you.

Safety precautions between people with CF did not always exist. Before cross contamination between individuals with CF was understood, intermingling was encouraged as a way for people to deal with the long loneliness that can be created by carrying a burden that only you understand. Tessa Weber, who grew up in Minnesota and now lives in a suburb of Boston, Massachusetts, remembers going to CF camp when she was fourteen. "I went to CF camp right before it shut down. That was a wonderful experience that was life-changing. I was very fortunate that I was able to go because you started to really learn about your body and what you're taking," she recalled. I imagine the feeling was like Talia's short encounter in the waiting room. You begin to learn, not only about other people, but more about yourself through meeting another person. "You start to feel you have some agency over your body a bit," Tessa explained.

Stephen Walter, who lives in the UK, remembers traveling with friends who had CF when he was a child: "When I was younger and before the realization about cross contamination and passing the bugs, we all used to go on holiday together. We [would] come back, and we'd all been really ill, and the doctors and nurses were scratching their heads." Around that time, research was occurring to see if there was a risk of close proximity. "All of a sudden it was, no, you can't see each other anymore. That support group of when I was younger, just chatting with other kids that had the same thing, suddenly just went," Stephen reflected. I can only imagine having a close group of friends and suddenly being told that because they are like you, you can never see them again. It would be especially heartbreaking in an era before the Internet and smartphones. Stephen tried to keep tabs on these friends but reflected that many had died. Never getting to say goodbye would not only be sad, but anxiety-inducing when you hear that your friend died, especially if they had the same disease as you.

Someone who has researched the transition of CF proximity is Becca Mueller. Becca was drawn to this topic because of her own CF experience. Her dissertation, "The Genome and the Biome: Cystic Fibrosis @ 6 Feet Apart," at the University of Pennsylvania in 2021, thoughtfully explores this transition through research and interviews. At a CF camp in 1989, an important breakthrough occurred—the realization that cepacia (a bacteria that causes swift deterioration of the lungs and is often fatal) can be transmitted between two patients. Through testing, scientists determined that the second patient had gained cepacia from another camper. Becca writes, "Though questions remained about the behaviors and host traits that led to transmission, [John] LiPuma and colleagues were certain that patient-to-patient spread had occurred."[31] Sputum cultures from children returning from other CF camps were analyzed to understand if the spread was occurring through physical proximity. Becca explains, "In the summers of 1987 and 1990, researchers studied the sputum cultures and social interaction of campers at sites in Michigan, Ohio, Utah, and Ontario. LiPuma was one of several dozens of co-authors of a report published in the June 18, 1993 issue of the *Morbidity and Mortality Week Report*."[32] Although these reports did not cause the immediate closing of CF camps, they influenced future proximity guidelines. Becca explains,

> The Morbidity and Mortality Weekly Report on transmission of cepacia at CF summer camps was only the beginning of epidemiologic work leveraging increasingly sophisticated molecular methods to study the identity and transmission of CF bugs. But looking back, the report did mark the beginning of the end of a certain version of CF sociality,

---

31. Rebecca Mueller, "The Genome and the Biome: Cystic Fibrosis @ 6 Feet Apart" (Unpublished Dissertation, University of Pennsylvania, 2021), 31.
32. Mueller, "The Genome and the Biome," 32.

one that was unfettered by infectious risk, where summer cabins, snacks, and kisses were shared without fear or self-consciousness. Although many questions remained about the integrity of the data and the appropriate policies to mitigate spread, the safety of the CF community became the subject of debate and the object of terror.[33]

Becca wrote her dissertation, in part, because she was interested in the way the CF community is fractured by the cross contamination issue. She explained, "As a clinician . . . I became very interested in that question of how this risk [being near other people with CF] was worth taking . . . and I found it really fascinating to understand the ways in which our community was broken up." Becca is grateful for Zoom "because it is a conduit for people with CF." She hopes to continue her research and to publish her dissertation, which would be a great gift to the CF community.

CF proximity guidelines became more widely known with the movie *Five Feet Apart*. Released in 2019, and starring Haley Lu Richardson and Cole Sprouse, the movie is inspired by the experiences of Claire Wineland, who died from CF in 2018. Although the film received mixed reviews from the CF community, it succeeded in raising awareness about CF. The film is not perfect, but the stress on isolation, as well as the effects of such isolation, is a moving aspect of the film. The title of the movie is based on Stella's desire to take back one foot of the six feet that CF protocols state she must keep from her new love interest, Will. Since both have CF, and Will has B. cepacia, Stella must stay away from him to prevent her from contracting the same bug and becoming ineligible for a lung transplant. The movie follows their emotional rollercoaster of dealing with their feelings and frustrations at not being able to be closer without risking their lives. Will's negative views toward relationships ultimately dissipate, as his protective "tough guy" mentality softens. I could easily understand his perspective and

33. Mueller, "The Genome and the Biome," 35.

pessimism about life and love. While the hospital setting of the movie bends its realism, the emotional toll of separation and loss is authentic. They have not only lost "one foot," but have lost the ability to be with the only people who might understand them. When viewed as a story of loneliness and isolation, I think the movie succeeds, far more than as a doomed love story.

The experience of navigating CF proximity with groups of people in *Five Feet Apart* is not only a storytelling device. Eliza reflected on how difficult it can be to navigate knowing someone else has CF while trying to respect when they don't want their diagnosis public. She had a friend in college who was less outspoken about having CF. Eliza reflected, "So, we had a quiet arrangement. Back then it was three feet apart. When we were in a room together, we would be three feet apart and nobody would need to know why." The two could share a glance and know that for safety's sake, they should keep their distance.

At one institution where I was teaching, I informed a colleague that I had CF. A few days later, she asked if I knew this student who also had CF. Upon receiving permission from the student, she gave me his name. Luckily, he was not a student in my class. I immediately reached out to him. We met in one of the classrooms, sat on opposite sides of the room, and briefly discussed what our lives were like with CF. We agreed to be extra careful about our proximity, like Eliza and her classmate. This was the first time I had a lengthy conversation with someone who also had CF. I felt like Talia when she met another person with CF in the waiting room. It was like meeting someone who was mythical. It also gave me a sense of fear. What if I had had him in class and he sat in the front row? What if this teacher did not learn that he, or I, had CF? My health was much worse than his, and I could have spread my bacteria to him, changing the trajectory of his life forever.

Following this encounter, I began to reflect on other encounters with people over the years. What if I didn't know someone else has CF? While many people with CF have a cough, some have gastrointestinal issues or other health concerns, or no issues at all. What if I were sitting next to a person on an airplane who had

CF? Even if the person is coughing, I am not going to suddenly demand to know if they have a chronic disease. We could travel for hours sitting next to each other, exchanging germs, less than six feet apart. This experience could be deadly for one of us and there is no way to know. Like some strains of COVID-19, you may never know if you infected someone and ultimately contributed to the death of a stranger.

Chase Honeycutt's insights about the CF World of isolation bring the concepts of vulnerability, loneliness, and community together. For his first seventeen years, Chase was able to avoid telling people he had CF. He recalls, "I had become very good at hiding CF. . . . Not even my good friends had any idea." When he got sick following high school, his life changed. "Having to explain why I had to go into the hospital for two weeks was a new hurdle for me . . . and that was the first time I had to sit and think about my illness," he confided. Over the next few years, Chase learned how dangerous it can be to have CF and how quickly one can go from seemingly healthy to being in the hospital.

In college, Chase attempted to hide his condition from others, just like Talia and me. "I tried so hard to hide that suitcase of meds . . . [I'd] put it in the closet and forget about it. Or [have] to run back to my dorm [to] not take my meds in front of people," he admitted. "And I felt very lonely in college because I didn't know anyone else with CF," Chase recalled, expressing his own sense of Dorothy Day's long loneliness. He began to sacrifice doing his treatments to hide his condition, which only made his health worse. "I was so convinced that my two worlds of having a social life and having a disease couldn't mix. . . . Much of my early life was spent trying to hide my own disease," Chase explained, echoing my CF journey.

When he was hospitalized during college, Chase still had not met or talked to anyone else with CF. He felt like he was fighting his battle alone. He reflected, "It [feels] like I'm the only person fighting this. Friends . . . visit . . . and they don't understand. It is hard to convey that you are terrified of something when you look healthy." Chase began to realize that frequent hospitalizations could become his new normal. He also had to come to terms with not knowing anyone else with CF: "All CF patients are isolated at the doctor's office. . . . So I still don't see anyone [who] looks like me, and it is weird." With the advent of social media, Chase now has reached out to people for support, but those experiences of isolation made an impact on how he grew into understanding what it means to have CF. He felt he had to hide his true self for so many years and is now slowly opening up to others.

At the conclusion of our conversation, Chase said, "This was, I guess, the first time for me, I've been able to openly talk about my experience. I appreciate it." His honest reaction touched upon an emotion for both of us. He was not the first person who expressed gratitude, at the conclusion of our Zoom conversation, for processing the CF experience with another person with CF for the first time. I never thought, when I began the project, that it would serve as a bridge for me and so many others—a bridge that connected an archipelago separated by the seas of the long loneliness, an opportunity to touch upon an emotion, even if physical touch within the community is forbidden, and a chance for Dorothy Day's prophetic voice to echo again: "We have all known the long loneliness, and we have learned that the only solution is love, and that love comes from community."

Conclusion

Garden Empathy

Entering the rose garden can be a scary place, especially when what you hear reflects something in your story. Limited time, medical struggles, and loneliness are spiritual realities that transcend race, religion, culture, and chronic conditions. They are human experiences. Part One has primarily explored life through the eyes of those with a chronic illness. These stories embody what it means to live "extravagantly" with CF, as people told their stories joyfully. That does not mean the content was always happy, but that people shared vulnerable parts of their lives so that you could touch something in their story, and, perhaps, touch your own.

Martin Tallant offers a way to bring together CF Time, CF Space, and CF World. He lives in the UK and was diagnosed with CF at the age of fourteen. Martin was hospitalized four times per year in his twenties, a time when "the damage has been done" to his body through repeated hospitalizations. In light of these experiences, he thoughtfully stated,

> If you take a child who is two or three years old and he is spending a ton of time in the hospital, and they see someone else who is the same age in hospital, all they want to do is interact with each other. They don't [care] about any other bit. Any kind of bigotry and racism has got no place in their world. They are just so grateful to socialize. And it makes their stay in the hospital so much easier. It does wonders for their mental health, as well. And it's one of those things that I'd say is, you know, I have been there, and I have been really unwell,

you know, not being able to get out for a couple of weeks. Anytime there is someone else there who knows how you are feeling because they are going through similar stuff. You don't [care] if they are gay or straight. If they identify as a . . . tree. You go, I'm really glad that you are here. Thank you for having a conversation with me. . . . Everyone is deserving of empathy and respect.

When two people share the same hospital room, they may watch the movement of the second hand together. These people may share the experience of doing everything they can to stay healthy, knowing these efforts will fall short. And those two people may agree that no one will understand them because illness isolates people. They may be grateful for any human being who will listen to their story. In the world of chronic illness, barriers that are often erected between people become very thin and may disappear. As a chaplain, my identity as a cis-gendered, straight, Catholic, white, middle-class man is less of a barrier for those who identify differently than it is in other places in society. It is my willingness to sit, listen, pray, and potentially to shed a tear that is important when a patient extends an offer to sit at their bedside. Having CF helped me understand aspects of this phenomenon before I began studying chaplaincy, and I suspect it is one of the reasons that I felt called to spend fifteen months doing this work. I wanted to offer my experience as one of the roses to help others.

Martin believes having CF taught him empathy. He reflected on his father and a good friend with whom he disagreed on nearly everything. At his father's funeral, this person gave the eulogy. Martin recalled, "Part of the eulogy was that this guy and my father were pretty much polar opposites . . . but they still enjoyed a pint. They still enjoyed each other's company." Martin sees this appreciation of difference as a powerful lesson for a world that is so divided and against listening to people with different views. He offered, "We should all be looking to learn from people we have disagreements with because it expands us." When you spend a lot of time with people who are alike in at least one way—they are confined to a hospital—you learn to listen, even if the person is very different in other ways. Martin explained that if he and a friend have a disagreement, they try to acknowledge it, "and then go, alright, we're getting a bit touchy. Now, let's just pull back, have a cup of tea, and put football on." I agree, Martin. If only others would listen when the roses speak.

Part Two

Pruning the Roses

L iving with a chronic illness is a helpful framework for approaching the revolutionary transformation of gene modulators. For those in the CF community who have benefited from them, the lens through which they view CF Time, CF Space, and CF World may be very different. Part Two attempts to capture how that worldview can be turned on its head and how such a reversal may affect an individual. Some describe this as having a whole new body or their old body finally functioning as designed. These treatments hold promise beyond treating cystic fibrosis. Bijal Trivedi says, in *Breath from Salt*, "I realized, the lessons of cystic fibrosis could be meaningful to millions—saving individuals suffering both from rare diseases, like Duchenne muscular dystrophy, and common ones, like cancer and Alzheimer's."[34] Those with other chronic illnesses who saw themselves or their loved ones in Part One may soon write their own Part Two transformation narrative because of gene modulators.

Pruning a rose means removing dead or diseased growth to help a flower grow. For many in Part Two, the pruning may be experienced as removing aspects of their CF experience that moved them closer to death—constant coughing, clogged airways, debilitating digestive issues—and replacing them with healthier movements of the mucus in their bodies. Just as a rose loses dead petals, those who have had positive experiences with gene modulators shed some of the most harmful aspects of the disease. The level of this improvement

---

34. Bijal Trivedi, *Breath from Salt: A Deadly Genetic Disease, a New Era in Science, and the Patients and Families Who Changed Medicine Forever* (BenBella Books, 2020), XVIII.

differs from person to person, just as CF manifests itself differently from person to person. You will find in Part Two a scent of joy from these roses, many who thought that falling to the ground "foil by foil" was near. Thanks to gene modulators, they will continue to grow and make the world beautiful for longer than many expected.

Chapter 4

The Rubicon

As expected, my PFT was low. I just started a new job and don't want to commit to IVs just yet. I am going to take some oral antibiotics for four weeks to see what happens. Somehow, that isn't even the worst news from my clinic visit today. The doctor mentioned before I left that at my next visit, I should meet with people to talk about the lung transplant process. I have been dreading this moment ever since I read about Mr. Luedeke in high school. My time has come. I don't know if I want to go through the process, but I don't want to "give up" because I know that will hurt my parents. I am scared and I don't know what to do. I am ok with not living, but I am also afraid to die. Good night.

Medical drugs do not appear willy-nilly on the market. They undergo years of research, multiple phase trials, and various reviews to determine if they are safe. There have been many developments in CF care that are described in detail by Bijal Trivedi in *Breath from Salt*. While these trials are important, the individual experience of those who have (or do not have) and lose (or gain) the medication during trials is rarely discussed in the arena of ethics. The experience of having a lung transplant adds a dimension to CF care. The notion of a gene modulator as a possible "cure" for CF means something very different for those who needed a transplant before access to a gene modulator could help them. The origin of the story of CF during the era of gene modulators is an important starting point for grasping the transformation that followed.

The Ethics of Progress

On October 19, 2011, Vertex Pharmaceuticals applied to the FDA for approval for a drug that would soon be named Kalydeco.[35] Trivedi explains, "The data was indisputable, the disease severe, and there was no other drug on the market to treat it. Patients were desperate; many were dying."[36] The approval came on January 31, 2012, in one of the fastest drug approvals in FDA history.[37] Not only was this medication a breakthrough for the 4 percent of the CF population who could take it, but it was also the beginning of a new approach to curing disease. Trivedi writes, "This was the first drug ever developed to treat patients with a specific genetic mutation. . . . It was the beginning of the personalized medicine revolution. . . . Now it [CF] was the first [disease] to have a medicine capable of targeting the root of the disease."[38]

Emily Schaller participated in the Kalydeco trials that helped make this FDA approval possible.[39] In 2009, she was told by a CF researcher about the trial. The person explained, "It's out of Cleveland, and you will have to drive there every seven days for three to six months, but it treats the mutation you have." Emily was sold. For months, she traveled from Detroit to Cleveland to be subjected to "crazy testing, like shoving tubes up my nose and running liquid through it to test the electrical charge in my sinuses." During this time, Emily felt no change and began to lose heart. "I'm doing all this testing and not feeling any better. . . . It's just a pill. What pill is going to do anything for you?" Emily decried. Soon after this trial, she got sick, causing her to assume this potential drug would not be as good as people hoped.

A short time later, she was enrolled in phase three of the trial, at the University of Michigan. She began a few days before Christmas, in 2012. "Within four days of taking this drug, I was a different

---

35. Trivedi, *Breath from Salt,* 417.
36. Trivedi, *Breath from Salt,* 417.
37. Trivedi, *Breath from Salt,* 420.
38. Trivedi, *Breath from Salt,* 421.
39. Emily's *Rock CF* organization was discussed in chapter 2.

person," Emily reflected. While spending time with her brother, she started laughing and realized something was different: "That laugh didn't turn into a coughing fit that needed a ten-minute recovery [like usual]. We just looked at each other and were like, What?" Her voice changed and her PFT skyrocketed. Her ability to run was transformed. "It feels like somebody flipped a switch on the back of my head. And things changed. And I could breathe," she said emotionally.

In 2012, few people knew of the transformative power of Kalydeco. Far fewer people were eligible to take it, and social media as it is now did not exist. "This little blue pill completely changed my life, and it was hard to talk about it with people because I was in the 4– 6% that could take it," she explained. Trying to tell people with CF, who have lived their whole life critically ill, that a pill would dramatically improve their health was challenging. Emily still takes Kalydeco, and through *Rock CF* she went on to become a champion for the cause of running and exercise to help keep people with CF healthy. However, a gene modulator that worked for other CF mutations was still years away.

On July 2, 2015, the FDA approved a second gene modulator from Vertex, which came to be known as Orkambi. This drug targeted those having two copies of the F508Delta mutation. It is estimated that just under 50 percent of the people with CF in the US were genetically eligible to take Orkambi. Clearly a much wider reach than Kalydeco, Orkambi represented the potential for progress for gene modulators. Trivedi describes that during the Orkambi Phase 3 trials, "After just six months, patients had fewer lung infections and fewer hospitalizations, and had begun gaining weight."[40] Unlike Kalydeco, however, the increase in lung function was not found to be 12%, but 2– 4%.[41] Those with CF and their families were still elated at the possibility of having something that could improve the lives of those with F508Delta, even if the lung function improvement appeared marginal.

---

40. Trivedi, *Breath from Salt,* 450.
41. Trivedi, *Breath from Salt,* 450.

I remember taking my first dose of Orkambi in 2016. I held the pill in my hand and wondered what it would do to me. At this point, my health was in decline, but I was still able to run multiple times a week. Despite losing 3–5% of my lung function per year and doing IVs approximately once a year, my health was decent. I wondered if there would be any negative side effects or if I would feel anything. I do not remember any serious improvement from Orkambi, but I do remember having a bit more energy and recovering from running more quickly. In 2016, I was able to complete my only full marathon in just under six hours; Orkambi likely helped me accomplish that feat. I remained on it for a few years and continued to need IV medication at the same frequency.

Maddie Core felt huge improvements with Orkambi, which she also began taking in 2016.[42] "That definitely impacted my life in a lot of ways," she recalled. "Before Orkambi, it was miserable getting up in the morning. I would just lay there for an hour or two because I dreaded getting up and having to cough everything up, . . . or when I was playing basketball with my friends, I couldn't keep up." But when she took Orkambi, everything changed: "I'd wake up and have nothing to cough up. And I could keep up with my friends." For Maddie, Orkambi was the drug that brought the miraculous change, just as Kalydeco did for Emily.

In 2018, Vertex's gene modulator, Symdeko, was approved. Symdeko was similar to Orkambi but was hoped to have fewer side effects, such as chest tightening.[43] Lizzie Whitla, who lives in Tasmania, has been taking Symdeko for the past three years. When she was thirty-one, she had to be hospitalized for a CF exacerbation, and after fourteen days in the hospital, she still wasn't feeling much better. "A month later, I got a call from our CF medical team that said I fit the criteria for Symdeko," she explained. Starting it made a huge difference: "I just went gangbusters from there. . . . It has kept me at a real steady level . . . and kept me out of the hospital." She has had negative effects with other gene modulators, but not

---

42. Maddie's experiences with CF friendships were discussed in chapter 3.
43. Trivedi, *Breath from Salt*, 463.

from Symdeko, again demonstrating how CF manifests uniquely in each person.

While trials were occurring for Orkambi and Symdeko, the most promising of the modulators was also undergoing trials. This drug, Trikafta, was different because it combined three different medications, elexacaftor, tezacaftor, and ivacaftor. The goal was to have a drug similar to Kalydeco in its effectiveness but targeting more of the CF population than Orkambi and Symdeko. The expectations that this new drug would accomplish this feat grew as it advanced through trials.

In October 2018, Zack Swanborn began the Trikafta trials but saw no change in his condition.[44] He reflected on his state of mind: "Oh my gosh, all of this hype, all of this research, and I am still getting sick. This is never going to get better." What had built up his hopes became another empty promise. In April 2019, the rollover from the study allowed him to get access to Trikafta six to eight months before other people. By this time, his baseline for PFTs had dropped to 60%. Zack immediately realized he was given the placebo during his early tests because his body's reaction to the medication was almost instant. Zack described, "Within forty to seventy-two hours I was noticing a huge difference. When I would laugh, I would just hack and hack and hack, . . . and I noticed when I was with some buddies that I was not coughing. . . . This is insane."

While Zack's medication was a placebo, Eliza Callard's experience was the opposite.[45] She got on the toxicity trial for Trikafta and immediately had amazing results. Unfortunately, she was only on the medication for one month at this stage of the study, and then it was taken away from her for a year. Eliza recalls, "And the change was so radical. And then I had a whole year before I was put back on the study. And I got really, really sick during that time. And I just didn't have much hope." Eliza had access to a drug that seemed to

44. Zack described the difficulty of navigating high school while adhering to medical treatments in chapter 3.
45. Eliza's relationship with her partner was described in chapter 3 in her desire to take a chance on love.

help her but had to wait nearly a year until the study was complete to have access to it again.

A third perspective on Trikafta trials is Rachael Russell's.[46] Rachael was on the phase two trial and knew she had Trikafta, rather than a placebo, like Zack, because of the amazing changes in how she felt. She took the experimental medication for three months. When she moved to phase three, she did not receive the medication; instead, she was given a placebo. "Being taken off of it so quickly my lung function just went down, down, down," she explained. Although it was a blind study, Rachael easily knew when she was on it and when she had the placebo. "I have lived with this my whole life. I know what to expect month to month," she explained. Going from being on it to having it taken away was very difficult: "It felt really unethical. . . . I understand they were still gathering data, but I had a 20% increase [in PFT] in the first month of taking it." Rachael powerfully explained that the loss was so difficult because "I [now] know how I should feel. I was healthy, this was life-changing, and you just took it away from me and I only have it for a couple of months. It was heartbreaking."

Drug trials are very important, and new medications need to undergo rigorous testing. Unfortunately, the experiences of people who are on trials are often forgotten. Zack began with a placebo and believed the most anticipated CF medication ever was useless (until he realized he had had the placebo). Eliza had an amazing result for one month, only to have to wait nearly a year to regain access. Similarly, Rachael went from a year of the medication to a placebo. Her chance at a more "normal" life was stuck in limbo as her body slingshot back to where it was before. Because the results of drug trials are often what makes headlines, it can be easy to forget that the people who undergo the trials experience physical and psychological side effects.

History records that when Julius Caesar led his army across the Rubicon he proclaimed, *alea icatc est,* or the die is cast. His decision ushered in a civil war. In modern parlance, crossing the

---

46. Rachael's experience with PFTs and compliance were described in chapter 2.

Rubicon insinuates there is no turning back. An action has been taken and has set things in motion. As I reflect on the development of gene modulators, this image comes to mind. CF care has changed dramatically. What was once a uniform group of sufferers has been split apart by gene type. Whether or not one can benefit from Kalydeco, Orkambi, Symdeko, or Trikafta, one thing is clear. CF care has changed. The die has been cast.

The Trade

While the drug trials of gene modulators pushed forward and people with CF waited with bated breath to see if their lives would be transformed, others realized that whatever might come about from this research would not be in time to help them. The day I read about Mr. Luedeke, I learned that the inevitable choice for many with CF would eventually become whether or not to have a lung transplant. In the 1990s, transplant success was less likely than in 2019, which is when I had the CF clinic visit described in the opening chapter's diary entry. Despite an increased success rate, I wasn't sure that I wanted a transplant. I had been taking Orkambi for a few years to slow my decline, but my lungs were now losing their capacity as my PFT neared 40%. Its descent toward 30% in 2020 became a foregone conclusion. This physical loss engendered a mental and emotional loss. I did not know if I cared enough to live. However, I knew I couldn't look my parents in the eye and tell them I wouldn't at least try to stay alive. It was an unenviable position.

Kassandra Klemenz, who currently lives in Knoxville, Tennessee, faced similar questions about having a lung transplant. Healthy and active in her younger life, she became very sick in her twenties. Antibiotics were no longer able to treat her lung infections. "It eventually deteriorated my lungs," she reflected. She moved from Tennessee to Massachusetts hoping insurance could cover a potential transplant. She soon found herself sick and in the hospital: "At first, I was against it [the transplant]. And I just wanted to [die]." But she found herself thinking about her possibilities in life and the opportunity to have more time with her partner Kevin. She reflected, "If I could have a life like that, even for a few years, it would be worth it."

Kassandra was in the hospital for three months awaiting compatible lungs. On January 6, 2020, her lung function was down to 8% and she was intubated. The same day the decision was made to let her die peacefully, new lungs arrived; Kassandra had the chance for a new life. The procedure was successful. Kassandra reflected with a smile, "Now that I have new lungs, I have never breathed this well. And I can tell [there is] a huge difference in everything that I do." At age twenty-three, she runs fifty miles weekly, swims regularly, and trains for triathlons. All things she never thought she would do as she was preparing to die.

Justin Goldsmith, who is married and lives in New York, also understands what it is like to weigh the pros and cons of a transplant. At age thirty-one, he had a very difficult discussion with his doctor concerning his health decline. "After that doctor's appointment, I went home. I cried a lot. I called my boss and stopped working then and there." His health remained steady enough until he was thirty-seven, and he needed the transplant. Following the procedure, he was told that the lung donor's family had made the decision to take them off life support. Holding back tears, Justin explained, "That really hit me hard. This family had lost a family member and then literally gave me life. It still . . . chokes me up. It is so amazing. And it is a precious gift that means a lot to me." Justin pointed out that not all operations go as smoothly as his. There was another person in the recovery ward who Justin remembers having a horrible time with his new lungs. "He was always saying he couldn't breathe, [and] he couldn't eat; he felt like he wasn't breathing at all. I think about him every now and then." He realizes that that person could have been him or anyone else given the intense nature of the procedure. Justin's choice to get new lungs in 2017 has given him a chance for life and the possibility of a family.

Justin also reflected on the only other person he knew with CF. Her name was Amy, and they met at the CF clinic. They became friends on Facebook and were both faced with the possibility of a lung transplant around the same time. Unlike Justin, she chose not to go through with the procedure. "I think her words to me were, 'I don't want to trade one set of problems for another set of problems.' And that is completely understandable. You are rolling the dice either way," He paused for a moment and then added, "She is gone. She has been gone for several years now."

Unlike Justin or Kassandra, Katherine Russell had little time to prepare for her transplant. It happened very quickly due to a serious bout of pneumonia. "It was not on our radar at all," she said. Her surgery was an unconventional form of lung transplant that cut down the center of her sternum and used a technique called bronchial artery revascularization. She needed this because inflammation and bronchiomalacia made a traditional transplant impossible. On her twenty-second birthday, she received new lungs. It took a month for her to be able to walk again, and her recovery was long. "So much has to align for your transplant to be successful," she reflected. Katherine is especially grateful for the love of those around her, which helped her during her recovery.

Katherine explained that recovery is not only physical. It is also mental and emotional, as you come to terms with what has happened. She offered that the survival rate for living five years after a lung transplant is fifty-fifty. Katherine explained that this is one difference between the transplant experience and taking gene modulators: "A lot of people are taking Trikafta and getting all this hope. Okay, I can start thinking long-term. Whereas after the transplant I was like, okay, I have more time. . . . It's limited though. Once I beat that 50 percent, I started to feel more confident. Now that I am at eleven years, I am thinking long-term."

Caleigh Haber has received not one lung transplant, but two. She also suffers from CF-related GI complications. "It is difficult to determine whether my lung issues or gastrointestinal issues have been more severe," Caleigh explained. "While I've needed two double lung transplants, which clearly explains the severity of my lung disease, the focus and concern has consistently been on my GI health, and that has always been a significant burden." Growing up she was very healthy until around age eighteen, when her health swiftly declined. Difficult family dynamics exacerbated her health issues. "I moved out," she explained, "and that marked the beginning of a downward spiral. . . . My disease progressed at an alarming rate." Her CF care team declared her ineligible for a transplant because of what they deemed as her previous "noncompliance." This sent Caleigh even deeper into despair. "I was placed in hospice and sent home. It was devastating. . . . I had no hope and no motivation to keep fighting." She was on oxygen and a feeding tube and was losing the will to live. Caleigh credits her mother with giving her the desire to keep fighting and to "correct" the things pointed out by the clinic that would make her eligible for a transplant. "It took me a year and a half to prove my compliance. I was only twenty-one at the time. I learned a great deal about responsibility and how to care for myself," she admitted. Following her transplant, her lungs went into rejection. Within a few months, she fell from 70% lung function to 20%. "It felt as though the wind had been knocked out of me—I was utterly defeated." She moved to another clinic where providers were willing to do a second surgery. Caleigh's lungs have been relatively healthy since that time.

Caleigh views the transplant experience as essentially trading one set of health challenges for another, noting that a CF cure would not fully address the complexities faced by transplant recipients. "For those of us who have undergone lung transplants, a CF cure doesn't mean we can simply put our health issues behind us. . . . We will always be on anti-rejection and immunosuppressive medications, which come with their own lifelong complications. We won't benefit from gene modulators that could alter our lung function, and we live with the constant threat of organ rejection," she explained. The risk is especially high given all the medications she takes and how those can cause other organs to fail. While the trade of one disease for another was needed to survive, it separates those who have had lung transplants into another camp of the CF community. Such is the cost of staying alive for those who were too sick before modulators or who could not benefit from them.

Mr. Luedeke made this trade. Less than three months after I read about him, the rejection of his lungs caused his death on May 22,

1996. Luckily, Caleigh was able to get a second transplant before she met the same fate. It is important to recognize the courage of those who have a transplant, and how the trade of one disease for another is often overlooked, especially during the gene modulator era. I am not implying that those like Amy who chose not to have a transplant lack courage. Warrior mentality is unhelpful when used to shame people into doing things others think they *should* do, and it takes courage to decide when the fight is over. Kassandra was uncertain about having a transplant. I am not sure what I would have done. The decision is an individual's choice, often influenced by how many other health issues a person has and their likelihood of survival. In many cases, it can be a Hail Mary pass to extend life that could result in more pain and suffering. Before gene modulators, a transplant was the only way to extend life at the final stage, and those who chose it should be acknowledged for all they do to stay well each day. If Trikafta had not come out when it did, Mr. Luedeke's experience may have been my own.

Chapter 5

Jackpot

This morning, I took my first dose of Trikafta. I just got back from the gym with Sean, and I think I was able to jog for two minutes before I had to walk on the treadmill. I am surprised I was able to go that long. I'm not sure, but it felt different. Maybe it is a placebo effect since it can't possibly be this new medication, can it? Nothing works that fast. I told Sean I would like to go back tomorrow. Since it is January 1st, I can start the new year off with another short run. Maybe 2020 won't be as bad as I thought! Let's see how I feel tomorrow. Good night!

It is not an exaggeration to state that Trikafta is a tremendous medical breakthrough. This chapter could be a book of transformation stories, which was my initial intent. Many of the people you met in Part One experienced a powerful transformation as well, but space limits how many stories I can share. These stories are divided into two groups: First, those who were approaching death, to illustrate the radicality of the medication. The second set highlights some new opportunities people have in a future they never anticipated, including the opportunity to have children.

From the Brink of Death

I remember the first time that, as a chaplain, I was called to the bedside of a person who was dying. It was my first solo evening shift at my internship at the Cleveland Clinic and I was terrified.

I was told that the doctor had been asked to remove life-sustaining measures and that the family of over ten people wanted to have a prayer said at her bedside. My hands were shaking as I rode the elevator up to the ICU. I thought, "Who am I to be doing this?" As I stood at the foot of the patient's bed and prayed, part of me hoped for a miracle. I thought perhaps my prayer would bring this elderly woman out of her coma. When I opened my eyes, however, no miracle had happened. She did not sit up. The weeping family thanked me as I stepped to the back of the room. As I returned to my office, I felt ill-prepared for the moment and wished something miraculous had occurred. I slowly learned that when people are in their final days or hours of life, it isn't likely they will recover. That happens in movies. In the hospital, these people die. The woman I prayed over left this world about two hours after I stood at her bedside and hoped for a miracle.

For those who work in the medical profession, this is their reality day after day. Especially in the ICU, where the sickest patients receive care, death is expected when a patient reaches a certain level of decline. That does not mean people do not recover in ICU, and it doesn't mean there are no unforeseen medical reversals where people live longer than expected. Indeed, the power of positive thinking, love of family, and perhaps prayer can have unexpected consequences. Recovery from near death usually takes a toll on one's body, and the older the patient is, the less of their previous quality of life is present. With that said, when a family gives permission for a patient to be put on CMO, it means death is likely near.

Like some of the patients I met in the ICU, Mason Williams was not sure how much time he had left to live. Growing up in Wales, Mason loved music but reasoned that his medical condition would prevent him from pursuing his dreams. By eighteen years old, he needed to be on oxygen overnight. Mason describes that being on oxygen so young "hit me and my family kind of hard." When he was twenty-one, he needed oxygen during the day. He carried the oxygen tank on his back and found himself in a wheelchair for days at a time. When he had a lung collapse in 2019, his CF team in London put in motion the process for a double lung transplant.

At the start of 2020, he was put on the urgent list, signaling that his transplant could be soon. Like the patients I have seen in the ICU, his condition was worsening, and without a lung transplant, he knew he did not have long to live. He was in the final stages of his life in his early twenties. His hopes of being a musician felt increasingly distant, as his lungs labored for each breath.

Mason had heard of Trikafta and "begged and pleaded with doctors" to hold off the transplant. "My family and I have known about this drug. . . . At least let me try it," he implored. On February 6th there was a knock on his hospital door. "We have got it! It is here!" his doctors exclaimed. "I started it. Within twelve to twenty-four hours, I felt cured. Completely cured," Mason emotionally reflected. Soon after starting Trikafta, he could walk in the hospital without gasping for air and he came off oxygen. After leaving the hospital he could freely take walks with friends and travel on weekends. Looking back, Mason affirmed that his CF decline "has halted. Completely frozen in its tracks." He returned to a sense of "normal" for a healthy person with CF.

For those with other chronic conditions, Mason's story may sound unbelievable. To go from a few months from death, without a transplant, to feeling "cured" is not only unlikely but borders on the "miraculous." A young man on oxygen and wheelchair-bound, preparing how he will spend his final days, leaves the hospital and no longer needs oxygen because of the efficacy of a few pills. Additionally, he can affirm years later that his health has been maintained. Organ transplants and aggressive forms of therapy may replicate such a turnaround, but these procedures carry other risks and complications that may lead to immediate death. For Mason, the side effects have been minimal. The primary effects have been transformative. He has backed away from the brink of death.

When I was six, my parents and I vacationed in Bermuda, not long after hurricane Emily had caused widespread devastation on the island and the ocean currents were still quite strong. On the first day on the island, my father took me into the ocean up to his knees. He was holding my hand when a huge wave struck us. I remember being underwater, not knowing which way was up. I tried to take a breath and began flailing my arms. The salt hit the inside of my mouth and panic ensued. I felt like a huge oceanic hand was pulling me by my ankles across the sandy bottom. I reached forward one more time hoping my father could get me. Then I felt his fingertips, followed by his other hand tightly grabbing my wrist. He pulled me up into his arms and he carried me back to shore. I began to cry, not sure if I was really safe. Since this episode, my father has recalled that he wasn't sure he was going to be able to get me, as he watched me being pulled out into the sea. This may be the closest I have come to the brink of death. The momentum was carrying me away, while his fingertips gave me life.

Like me in Bermuda, Mason was sinking. His lungs were filling as he gasped for air. The doctor's announcement of the arrival of Trikafta was like my father's fingertips, pulling us both to safety, where we could breathe fully. It was a final chance to be saved before being pulled under—one last opportunity to survive. The closer you are to death, the more surprising it is when the hand catches you.

Like Mason, Nick Laing's life was also saved by Trikafta.[47] Once Nick hit his teens, hospital admissions for lung issues became frequent. One year, he was admitted twelve times. "During my teen years, I was hardly ever at school because I was so sick," he reflected. His attendance made school a constant struggle. He spent much of his twelfth year being homeschooled. Doctors gave him a feeding tube, which still gives him nightmares. From October 2020 to October 2022, he had fourteen admissions and was listed on the transplant list for a double lung transplant. "My team was adamant that if my health continued to deteriorate as it had been . . . I would . . . die," he emotionally reflected.

Nick knew Trikafta existed in the US. A loved one in the US offered to try to pay for Trikafta, and one of his doctors encouraged him to start a process to get access to it. He also considered moving to Australia to gain access. While he was in the hospital, a box of Trikafta arrived. He does not know where it came from,

---

47. Nick's experience of being bullied as a child for having CF was described in chapter 3.

but he started taking it because he thought it was his only chance to live. "Within three hours of taking it, . . . [the effect] was pretty instant," he says describing the feelings of change. He took his first dose on October 4, 2022. Since then, he has gained a lot of weight, and his chest x-rays are "phenomenal". "My whole life has changed," Nick affirmed. New Zealand is currently funding his access to Trikafta.

Nick is able to work full-time and his PFT has gone up a lot from his lowest at 14%. He no longer coughs every thirty seconds. "I was so fearful [of] going to sleep at night. The minute I got up the next morning, everything in my chest would start moving and it would feel like there [was] a heavy blanket on it and I would cough for two hours. Then I would be too exhausted to do anything else," Nick explained. Now he doesn't cough at all at night. "The coughing, all of that is just gone," he reflected. "It's remarkable." Nick was featured in the *New Zealand Herald* for this amazing transformation, with the headline, *Miracle Drug Gives Bay Man New Life.* "My whole bucket list has changed. . . . I didn't think I would be around to see my twenty-second birthday. . . . If I could go back now and tell my twelve-year-old me that I would reach thirty-eight and life would be different, . . . my twelve-year-old self would be like, 'you're lying,'" Nick reflected. He now could have many more years than he ever expected.

"It . . . saved my life," Raelene Goody affirmed, echoing the transformation described by Mason and Nick. Raelene lives in England and was fairly healthy into her teenage years. She recalls learning about CF life expectancy while watching a TV show with her parents when she was around fifteen. This sent her into a spiral of depression requiring therapy. Following her teenage years, her lung function began to fall into the 30s, eventually down to 26%. Around the age of thirty-one, she was told that she needed a lung transplant and that she "should have been on oxygen a long time ago." "That really shocked us all," she confided. She began having anxiety while being on oxygen. "It was really difficult to walk and to go upstairs. . . . I would have a half-hour coughing fit," Raelene explained. Even waking up became a horrible experience, as one movement would wake up her body and then she would cough so much that she would be exhausted for the rest of the day. Any sense of quality of life was slowly slipping away.

When Raelene gained access to Trikafta, through Vertex's compassionate use program, her quality of life dramatically improved.[48] She does not think she would be alive today without it. She has been able to attend drama school and pursue her love of singing and acting. "It [school] is so intense, there is no way I would have been able to do a percentage of drama school without Trikafta," she reflected. However, Raelene is still processing that her lung function "only" rose to 33%. Although she is off oxygen and off the transplant list, she isn't as healthy as some people taking Trikafta. "It has been hard seeing so many people have increased lung function. . . . You compare yourself and you shouldn't," she confided. "I don't know if I will get that extra time. People can think about being an old lady, and I am not even sure I will get up to sixty," she confided. Her gratitude, despite this slight disappointment, was apparent. "It is just amazing," she reflected smiling.

Joshua Mitchell's brink of death was not only the debilitation of his lungs but also his mental health, as he considered taking his own life as his body deteriorated. Joshua grew up in the south of France and spent a lot of time on the ocean with his father, a sailor. He moved to Canada in 2010, and the change in climate greatly impacted his health. "I almost died when I was fourteen. I had a really bad case of pneumonia and was in the ICU for a month," he recollected. Joshua missed a lot of high school and barely graduated because he was so sick. His mental health began to decline as well. "I was angry at everything. It was . . . like, what's the point?"

By 2021, his health declined so much that he had "kind of given up." "I considered suicide many times, I was really depressed,"

---

48. This is also referred to as "expanded access" and is when a medication or vaccine is made accessible to those with a need deemed critical. The criteria for expanded access to Trikafta can be found on the Vertex website at https://www.vrtx.com/en-us/medicines/expanded-access/. Some who gained access to Trikafta in this book did so through this method.

he acknowledged. In November 2021, Joshua began crying on his morning commute. He recalls this particular morning as the "straw that broke the camel's back" of his decline. "Walking to work felt like I was working out," he explained. His job involved talking to customers, and he was constantly coughing in front of them. Joshua told his boss he no longer could continue, and that he had to step away. The many trips to the hospital throughout high school had taken their toll on his body. He lived alone and saw no options other than going on full financial aid. "I am not a lazy person. I love to work. I love being active," he affirmed. His body was taking away those things that he enjoyed.

A month later, Joshua began taking Trikafta and everything changed. "It felt instant," he described. Joshua soon got a full-time job at a restaurant and began exercising daily. He then enrolled in courses to begin a career he had always wanted—real estate and building development. Although he had always wanted to go down this path, he knew he would be too sick to practice by the time he got his license. "I [now] have a path. I have a blueprint," he asserted. Everything has changed. Joshua no longer pushes the heavy boulder of CF Space every day until he is exhausted. He no longer lives on the brink of death.

That first time I left the room of a dying patient I realized the stakes were high as a chaplain. Sometimes people expect a miracle and ask for a chaplain in the hopes that a prayer will cure their loved one. Death is far more likely than miracles in the hospital. Reflect, for a moment, if you know someone who has a chronic illness and how unlikely and powerful it would be if a pill removed most of the life-threatening manifestations of that illness. Those on oxygen could breathe on their own, those in wheelchairs could walk, those who cough constantly no longer cough, and those who have given up on life suddenly experience a dramatic turnaround, pulled from the undertow of the brink of death by a hand holding a few pills. Miraculous!

The Gift

While it is powerful to hear about Trikafta from the perspective of what it has held off (death) it is also insightful to look at the experience through what it has given (new life). Trikafta enabled Lori White to give a gift she never thought possible. "My mom and I made this pact when I was a young child that I was going to live longer [than her]," she said emotionally. Lori was born in 1972, at a time when living in CF Time often meant an early death; but her mother had hopes that Lori would be able to outlive her life expectancy. Lori was relatively healthy growing up, but in 2011 her condition began to decline. Her treatment regimen increased and so did the seriousness of infections. Her first hospital stay was in 2015, when she had double pneumonia, and she was put on oxygen and the lung transplant list. "I felt like this was it," she reflected. Her lung function had dropped to 19% and her weight was down to 93 pounds. She moved in with her mother, who saw how sick she was. They both feared the pact was not going to be able to hold up.

On November 7, 2019, Lori's life changed when she took her first dose of Trikafta. "It felt like somebody literally stretched open and added lungs to my lungs," she explained. The next day she told her wife, "I can feel air in my lungs. I can taste the air." Lori could go to a movie without her oxygen tank. "I realized, I don't cough anymore. What is going on?" she wondered. Lori and her partner recently bought a house because she sees the possibility of living long enough to enjoy it. Perhaps the most impactful component of her transformation was in her relationship with her mother. Her mom lived long enough to see her daughter have a chance to do the things in life she wanted to accomplish. "She was able to see me as a healthy person. I was able to give that to my mom because of Trikafta," Lori emotionally recalled. What a beautiful gift for her mother as she was dying, to know that her daughter would outlive her. The pact had been honored.

While Lori gave a gift to her mother, Emily Lawrence's Trikafta experience is a gift for her and her fiancé. Emily began college in the fall of 2019 and started Trikafta in November of that year. She noticed the changes immediately. "I always had problems coughing things up, even with the vest," she explained. With Trikafta she was able to clear her lungs. "My energy level is another thing I noticed," Emily said. She could now run errands and not have to go to bed immediately. "I went from sleeping all the time to bouncing off the walls," she recalled smiling. Her lung function had been down to the high 20s, and she was talking to doctors about transplants. Now she has a lung function in the 60s, the highest since 2015. "I swear, I felt like almost a completely different person," she affirmed. In thinking about the future with her fiancé, she explained, "We can plan for our future. We can sit back and take it slow. So that is definitely nice." Emily graduated in 2023, from the University of North Carolina at Charlotte, with a degree in social work. Instead of debating whether to set a wedding date before or after a transplant, Emily can think of her future, her career as a social worker, and the possibility of having a family. Her life is a gift she never expected.

Trikafta has given Marc Cotterill the gift of new time. Marc lives with his family in England and was one of the first people in the UK to receive Trikafta through compassionate use from Vertex. Before taking Trikafta, he would wake up every day in "exhausting coughing fits that would end with a severe headache," he described. With each passing year, he watched as his body deteriorated, despite trying to work out and remain healthy. His lung function slowly crept downward from the 40s into the 30s. He described the sensation as "drowning in his own flesh." "I was spending probably six hours a day on airway clearance alone," he recalls. He quit work in 2019, not knowing if he would ever be healthy enough to go back.

On March 3, 2020, Marc got a call that Trikafta was being shipped to his hospital. The nurse called and asked if he wanted to get it next week. "I'm in the car. I'm on my way," he responded. He took that dose immediately after she passed it to him through the window. Later that afternoon he began to feel different. "Like, all of a sudden, I was hydrated," he remarked. That evening he had the purge, and it was easy to bring up the mucus from his lungs.[49] The next day, he did not begin the day coughing and went for a run instead. "I think the most surprising thing was the speed," Marc expressed, concerning the changes his body experienced on Trikafta. "That very first moment, it was like waking up in a new body. It was the weirdest, most amazing experience. It felt like a second chance," he continued. "The biggest gift that Trikafta has given . . . it's given time—but not just time—quality time." Marc, and so many others, have been given a gift that cannot be repaid. If the greatest lie ever told is that you have time, perhaps the greatest gift one can be given is more time.

Alexa Ciancimino, who lives in Las Vegas, was also given an unexpected gift. She watched her lung function decline into the 70s during college, and then down to a baseline of 42% a few years later. She reflected on the difficulty of living in CF Space: "So it just kept dipping, frequent antibiotics, being in the hospital . . . that whole vicious cycle." During one admission her lung function was down to 20%. Her doctors told her, "Your lungs are terrible. You are really sick. If we can't get your lung function up, you will have to consider [a transplant]." Her lung function rose back to 38%, but she still experienced the up-and-down cycle. She was discouraged and afraid of what the future would bring.

On December 8, 2019, Alexa began Trikafta. She experienced a day or two of the purge and then woke up the next day to find her cough was gone. Her PFT is currently up to 70%. Smiling, she said, "I never expected that in my wildest dreams. There are just no words. It gives you your whole life back. Your life is going in one direction, and then it goes the complete opposite." She has not been sick, she doesn't cough, and she is amazed at these changes. Alexa thoughtfully offered a beautiful image of the unlikelihood of getting a life you never thought you could have: "It is like winning

---

49. The "purge" is a description that many people who took Trikafta used to explain the hours after taking Trikafta when their body "purged" itself of mucus. For some, it was a violent series of coughs lasting over an hour, coughing up more mucus than they ever had before.

the lottery." After years of struggle and wrestling with an early death, Alexa's CF manifestation was given the numbers 20-18-9-11-1-6-20-1 and hit the jackpot.[50] It is hard to imagine a better gift.

I would also use the word "gift" to explain my Trikafta experience. The diary entry for this chapter describes the first day I took Trikafta and my experience at the gym. I do not recall if I had the purge. I likely coughed more over multiple days, similar to Alexa. I knew little about Trikafta and likely thought I was just sick or coughing more, despite feeling like I could go a bit further on the treadmill. I don't remember the moment when I stopped having the constant cough. I suspect it slowly phased out. A few weeks after starting it, I was transcribing a recording of myself for a research project. I was coughing constantly on the recording, which made it hard to transcribe. I suddenly realized that I no longer coughed. I fought back tears as everything hit me. I had been given the gift of breath, the chance to breathe without coughing constantly. Eventually, I came to see the ramifications of this, when my PFT went from the low 40s to 55%. I couldn't believe it.

As I reflected more deeply on what this could mean for my life expectancy, I saw the gift, like Lori. Despite how bad my mental health had become by 2019, I continued to fight on because I could not imagine my parents having to bury their only son. I can now say it is likely they won't have to attend my funeral. The CF Time lens will always be part of me. However, I can now think a few years ahead. The boulder is a bit lighter, and I can go through my day free of the shackles of a dying body. I have not lost lung function since that initial post-Trikafta PFT. I may not live to retirement, but I am certain of one thing. I have lived far longer than I would have without Trikafta. I had the privilege of playing the lottery with Alexa and using the same numbers. I hit the jackpot too. These winnings will be more than enough to live on.

---

50. T-R-I-C-A-F-T-A!

The Baby Boom

I never wanted to be a parent. I am not sure if I felt this way before I learned that CF severely limited the likelihood that I could have a biological child. Perhaps I decided I didn't want to have kids after learning that it was unlikely I could, as a way of dealing with that reality. Or, maybe, learning that my life expectancy was thirty put me in a position where I knew I wouldn't see a child grow up, and therefore, I prepared myself by not wanting to be a parent at all. Some people with CF have similar views about having children instilled in them at an early age, while others mourn this loss and feel that something important has been taken from them. For some people, Trikafta has shifted the conversation around children.

"I've always been dead set against having children," expressed Annabelle Brown, who lives in England. Annabelle didn't think it would be fair to have a child and not live long enough to see a child grow up. She had her first IV treatment at thirteen, which marked the initial decline of her health. "And that was my first real, I suppose it sounds dramatic, but kind of experience of the fragility of life," she reflected. In September 2020, she gained access to Trikafta and experienced the purge. A few days later, she realized her sweat was no longer salty.[51] "I noticed I was . . . sweating like a normal person," she explained. Not long after, she realized Trikafta had affected her coughing as well. "Eventually, my cough just disappeared," Annabelle recollected.

These physical changes are not the only things that have changed in her life. Annabelle now has a different view on the possibility of having children. She reflected, "Now, I actually do want children because since taking Kaftrio,[52] it has . . . alleviated those pressures [of not seeing a child grow up]. And it has given me hope for a normal lifespan." "It makes me feel less guilty about ever having a family," she confided. Kaftrio has given Annabelle and her partner hope

---

51. People with CF sweat higher levels of chloride (one of two components that make up sodium chloride or NaCl).
52. The European brand name for Trikafta. It is the same drug.

for things that she never thought possible. Now it is far less likely that her potential future child would be left motherless because of cystic fibrosis.

Angela Oder is a CF nurse at the University of Cincinnati's CF Center. Angela came into CF care from palliative care three years ago when dramatic changes were taking place in the CF community due to gene modulators. She explained, "My expectation was that this patient population would be really ill. . . . When I transitioned over, modulators were really booming. I was surprised to see a majority of these patients doing really well. It was not what I expected." This change has come as a pleasant surprise. Another unexpected component of CF care, in light of gene modulators, has been the number of babies born to parents with CF. "When I think of Trikafta, I think of our baby boom," she reflected smiling. Angela thinks that a creative way to celebrate this achievement might be to post pictures of all the babies born to CF parents.

If this wall existed at Riley Aroche's CF clinic, her baby Siobhan would be on it. Prior to taking Trikafta in 2020, Riley lived her life expecting to be dead before she reached eighteen. CF affected Riley's ability to go to school, play sports, and hang out with friends. She never expected to go to college. Trikafta has allowed her to "do the things I didn't think I would be able to do before." Her lung function increased tremendously from a low of 23% into the 80s. Perhaps most surprisingly, after trying for years to have a child, she found out she was pregnant four months after taking Trikafta. "It was pretty shocking. . . . My doctors said one of the side effects could be getting pregnant right away," she recalled, acknowledging that she still did not expect it. Riley reflected: "[I'd] never thought I'd see the day when I wouldn't struggle to breath." Not only can she breathe, but her daughter Siobhan is alive and well. Trikafta has given Riley two lives she never expected: her own and her daughter's.

Morgan Barrett was also shocked when she discovered she was pregnant. Morgan and her husband had been married since 2015 and did not expect to be able to get pregnant. In December 2019, she began taking Trikafta. A few months later, she thought the changes in her body and her weight gain were part of the typical Trikafta increase until her mother offered that she should take a pregnancy test. "I'll do it just to humor you," Morgan told her mother, affirming, "I am not pregnant." She continued, "So I went into the bathroom, not expecting anything, looked at [the first test] and was like, wow. So, I did the [the second test] . . . and then told my husband." A visit to the doctor revealed that she was not only pregnant but was expecting twins. Looking back, she shared, "I thought, . . . I cannot imagine doing this with full-fledged CF. I can't imagine doing this before Trikafta; I don't think physically I would have been able to. It took so much out of me."

Morgan's Trikafta changes, like Riley's, transformed her life. A day after taking Trikafta, she was at the dentist and couldn't stop coughing. "I just felt so embarrassed," she recalled. When she got to her car, she realized there may be a connection between taking Trikafta and the uncontrollable purging in her lungs. Morgan describes a powerful moment that evening: "That night, I felt my lungs were so clear, clearer than they have ever been. Once I got everything up, I wasn't coughing anymore. And I remember it just felt cavernous. Oh my gosh, there is so much room and it doesn't hurt." Morgan's first adult breaths with clear lungs are a gift she never thought she would have—just like her children, Alder and Winslow. Someone who never thought she could be a biological mother could one day become a grandmother.

Jess Ragusa lives in Australia with her partner James. Before Trikafta, they considered IVF as a way of having a biological child together. Doctors told James, "You need to be prepared to raise this child by yourself. Jess isn't going to live for very long [due to CF]. She might not get very long into [the child's] life before she dies." Due to her health, Jess found the possibility of having a child with IVF a daunting task. In late 2021, before starting the IVF procedures, she began taking Trikafta and became pregnant without IVF. Jess recalls, "I felt like a whole new person instantly. Within twenty-four hours, my cough was gone." Before Trikafta, she had a very different idea of how her life would go. "I never thought I would be able to go to uni [university], buy a house, marry my husband, or have a baby," she explained. Her son Cooper is alive and thriving thanks to Jess taking Trikafta. "I couldn't imagine having a baby physically without Trikafta." Jess is now twenty-nine, and the life expectancy in CF Time given to her as a teenager was thirty. Jess said with a smile, "I hope to prove them [those who said she wouldn't see her child grow up] wrong."

The possibility of having a family is not only a new phenomenon for women with CF. Casey Bruce lives in Olympia, Washington with his wife and daughter, something he never expected. Echoing Annabelle's hesitations about having a child, Casey mused, "I just felt like it would be a little unfair. . . . I'm going to be a co-parent and then I'm going to need to check out before too long because I'm not going to live." He felt he would stick his wife with a mortgage, and she would have to raise a child on her own. "I just wouldn't feel right about that," he explained. Growing up, Casey's CF was mild. Like me, he remembers the moment when he learned the life expectancy. He discovered his grim prognosis as a teenager while watching a TV show with a character who has CF. Casey's health began to decline in his mid-twenties. In 2020, he contended with multiple infections and went into the ICU. He woke up from a coma three days later. Casey had been hospitalized for three weeks when he began Trikafta, in May 2020. It changed his life. His improvement was more gradual than for some people. After a few months, he "started to feel like he was really noticing huge improvements." After a year, Casey reflected, "I . . . felt like it was the healthiest I've felt in decades, . . . like the Trikafta had taken me back to a period . . . before I started to notice [CF]."

Seeing how much better he was doing on Trikafta, Casey said to his wife, "You know what, I think I'm ready. Let's do it." Their daughter is almost twenty months old, and Casey is so happy being a parent. "Being a dad is . . . my favorite thing I've ever done, " he said emotionally. "She is so great. I just love her so much and love spending time with her. It feels like a fantasy come true." Casey's joy toward having a daughter is so evident. There are many things CF can take from people. Casey's daughter Ivy will one day understand that without Trikafta, she never would have existed.

Eric Verdon lives with his wife in Canada. They recently married, after being together for eight years. Eric had previously hesitated to have children. "We had talked about having a family, and it's something I have always wanted," he explained, "but there is always the thought in the back of your mind. . . . What's the quality of life I am going to have?" Eric grew up playing sports and being active. If he had kids, he would want to play an active role in their lives. If he didn't have the energy to be with his children or had to spend that time in the hospital, what kind of father would he be? "Now, with Trikafta, a lot of those concerns are gone," he explained. His biggest health issue prior to Trikafta was coughing up blood and being hospitalized every eight months. "When I started Trikafta, the most notable thing for me was no hemoptysis," he expressed. In the past two years, he has not coughed up blood once, a transformation that he describes as "remarkable." His PFT is also remarkable, now at 115%. Eric's health transformation has invited him to rethink the question about what kind of father he could be, and because of Trikafta, he could be the kind who will live long enough to be active with his children and to see them grow up. Perhaps that is the most remarkable of it all.

Many who took Trikafta shared stories like these. Some who were "healthier" had fewer physical changes; however, they recognize CF as a debilitating disease and they are grateful to have access to it should they experience a steep decline. Other people's lives were dramatically transformed with incredible speed. In these cases, Trikafta was a life raft that saved them from the undertow, an unexpected life preserver fighting against the tide, a gift to themselves and those they love—with ramifications for generations who otherwise would never have lived. Jackpot!

Chapter 6

Who Is in the Mirror?

I was prepared to die. I had my affairs in order and had accomplished everything I wanted to do. I knew who I was and roughly how much time I had left. Now that I am taking Trikafta, I don't know who I am anymore. The past few years taking it have been amazing physically so why am I struggling psychologically? Shouldn't I be happy? There are many people who would do anything to hold those pills in their hands and here I am, struggling with things and seeming to complain when I feel better than I have in years. If anyone reads this, they may think me crazy, or suicidal, or ungrateful. I don't even know how to explain it to myself. I used to know who I was, but I don't anymore. After so many years of being "Jimmy who is dying" I don't know what it means to be "Jimmy who is living." Maybe I should rip out this page. No one would understand. Good night.

Pruning roses is not always easy. It means cutting things away and changing the flower's appearance. If the rose could talk, it might feel it is losing part of its essence. Whatever is cut away will change the rose and the way others see it. Life transformations do not come without a cost to one's identity, like the pruning of a rose. Many people struggle with change in their lives and how to adapt to something new. Yes, it is the same rose, but it could be significantly altered. Trikafta has left many with an altered sense of self and a new challenge. What does it mean to live as a person with CF whose manifestations of CF are greatly reduced? This chapter treats mental health questions from the perspective of the way an individual experiences the world.

The Midnight Sun

On February 6, 2023, the *New York Times* published an opinion guest essay entitled, "What It's Like to Learn You're Going to Live Longer than You Expected." The article was written by Daniela J. Lamas, a pulmonary and critical care physician at Brigham and Women's Hospital in Boston, Massachusetts. Much of the essay focuses on the experience of Molly Pam. Molly was approaching a lung transplant, just as I was, and then she began taking Trikafta. Now, her life and opportunities have been transformed. However, this transformation comes with a new set of questions about who she is and how she could live her life.

Lamas cites another physician at the same clinic, Dr. Manuela Ceradas, who states, "It's a tremendous blessing for most patients, but it can also be a source of anxiety. You had this thought of how your life would play out. It's what you were prepared for. But now you are going to live a lot longer. It can be a lot to go through. It can be a lot to process. What are you going to do with that time?"[53] The essay offers ways to live in CF Time by highlighting the decisions that some have made. It also points to the future, the possibility for cures for other terminal conditions, which could be just around the corner. Currently, incurable patients with numerous ailments may have their lifespans drastically increased. The experience of those battling CF and wrestling with a new lease on life may be a precursor to a question that will be faced by other people living with chronic and seemingly terminal medical conditions.

---

53. Daniela J. Lamas, "What It's Like to Learn You're Going to Live Longer than You Expected," *New York Times*, February 6, 2023. https://www.nytimes.com/2023/02/06/opinion/cystic-fibrosis-treatment.html

I would like to add an image to the metaphors of the second hand of a clock and Sisyphus pushing a boulder up a hill from Part One. When I began running and training for half-marathons, my athlete friends explained to me that when running a race, you hold back just enough to have a "kick" at the end. The final mile, half mile, or even the last portion of a race, should be when you explode with a burst of speed to try to finish as strong as possible. I think I was entering that metaphorical phase of my life. I was using everything I had to just get through the day. I knew I was only going to eke out a bit more. I could see the finish line, which symbolizes the finish of my life. I was "all in" and had accomplished everything I wanted. As I approached the finish line, it was as though I saw a sign boldly proclaiming, "This half-marathon has been changed to a full marathon, sponsored by your friendly medication, Trikafta." Wait, what? I just used my "kick" and was already mentally across the finish line. You just extended my race? I have nothing left [to do], so how [why] should I keep going? That is how I felt when I thought about this transformation. "Jimmy who is dying" was content with a half-marathon. "Jimmy who is living" was just told it is a full marathon. I didn't train for it; I didn't expect it, and I don't even know if I want it.

There was a time when I had a bucket list. Some of the things on it, such as finishing my dissertation or completing a full marathon (a real one), were eventually completed. Other things, like visiting Antarctica or all seven continents, were systematically removed from my bucket as my health worsened. By the fall of 2019, I made sure there was nothing left in the bucket. I had come to accept that I was dying and that the few years I had left would be spent trying to stay healthy enough to work. There was no time to think about dating, travel, or hobbies. I was in survival mode, mostly because I did not want to die before my parents.

By the end of the first week of January 2020, those identity markers were being erased. For those who have not been through the whiplash of this transformation, it may sound disingenuous that one would not fully embrace this gift. Those who are still waiting for access to Trikafta, or another new medication, may find it difficult to hear these statements. I hope it is clear that the reflections in this chapter do not take the gift of access to Trikafta for granted. However, the mental and physical changes that it causes in some people need to be considered, especially their mental health and personal identity. You can't really begin the work of processing this change of reality until you've arrived at that part of the race.

Monique Renee beautifully articulated her identity journey with Trikafta. By 2018, CF had an increased deleterious effect on her life. She was always sick and had to stop working. She accepted the fact that she would die young. Going to therapy helped Monique accept her seemingly inevitable decline. She explained, "I defined myself as the person who had this illness but is overcoming it and thriving, in spite of it." It doesn't mean she wasn't struggling as she slowly lost the ability to live a more dynamic life, but she was working to accept it. By the fall of 2019, her lung function was around 40%. A lung transplant was on the horizon, just as it was for me. "It was my biggest kind of fear, the transplant," she explained.

In November 2019, however, all of this changed. "Seemingly overnight it [CF] was gone," she said. The first day Monique took Trikafta, she was traveling with her partner. After driving for a few hours, she realized she had forgotten to do her morning treatment and that she was not coughing. "I broke down sobbing," she reflected. She was "completely overcome with emotion." She can now walk on the beach and keep up with her partner, go rock climbing, and go to a theme park without a wheelchair. She can have the life she never dreamed she could have again.

As people were confined to their homes during the pandemic, she began to think more deeply about all the changes she was experiencing: I began to ask myself, who am I? I don't recognize myself anymore." Monique felt a loss of community because she no longer identified with those who had a chronic illness. It sent her into a spiral: "Figuring out what was underneath CF was scary." Moving from survival mode to this new place was overwhelming. She was not prepared: "In some deep, dark place I was missing cystic fibrosis. This new life was scary."

Monique spent about a year working through these questions to figure out who she is post-Trikafta. She discovered new parts of herself, and she spent time exploring spirituality. "I pulled myself out of my identity crisis by finding new things to add to my identity," she explained. Once the fear of self-discovery wore off, it became exciting. Her therapist told her to try to go into new things with curiosity and encouraged her to embrace this new identity. It took time, but she now identifies herself as "Monique who is living."

Monique's observation that she was in some ways missing CF may sound odd, or privileged. It isn't that people want to be sick; it is that they knew who they were while sick, and now they need to rebuild their identity. For a person in their twenties, thirties, or forties, to be told you are starting over can be incredibly scary. It takes a lot of work to apply skills that may not have been developed or were severely altered by living in CF Time, CF Space, and CF World. Before gene modulators, many people were fighting in the present, waking each day to push the boulder uphill, only to deal with the emotional toll of watching it roll back down as they got sick again. It is possible to be grateful for the positive benefits of Trikafta while also mourning the loss of an important aspect of yourself.

Ben Mudge, an online coach in Belfast, echoed similar thoughts to Monique's about an individual's identity when on Trikafta. Ben was fairly strong growing up but described always having his future decline in the back of his mind. He explained growing up with CF as "someone chasing you, going the . . . same speed as you. They are always there." He also thinks that the impact of having CF on your mental health is often downplayed. "The mental health aspect of having something like this, it's just exhausting," he explained.

Ben didn't believe people taking Trikafta when they described it as breathing correctly for the first time, but only five hours after taking his first dose, he understood. Following his first dose, Ben stood at his sink and took a breath: "I felt my lower lung pop open . . . and hit my rib cage where I have never felt before, and I didn't cough. And I just burst into tears. . . . I thought, there is no way this is real." He can now laugh freely without altering his laugh for fear of coughing.

Ben and his wife were in disbelief about the speed of the change and what Ben was experiencing. Such a quick change can be difficult for anyone to process. Ben's transformation, and his opportunity to talk to other people with CF as a coach, have given him perspective on the radical change that Trikafta can engender. "It can feel like something has been taken from us. Part of your identity has been taken. You feel like you can't say that because we are extremely privileged to [have it]," he explained. Like Monique, Ben is trying to describe how one can mourn the loss of something that was always deemed bad, without denying the privilege of having a medication transform your life. Ben continued, "You have lost a section of your life, for the best reason, but now you . . . start thinking about things . . . you half believed in. Pensions, getting older, all those things that you . . . locked away in a box and you said, we will get to that, maybe, we will see." Few people can understand the tension of appreciation and confusion that comes with Trikafta. Talking to others who are wrestling with it can be a good support. Ben agrees: "When you speak to someone that you know has had those thoughts, even those [thoughts] you may be ashamed or don't want to announce to the world, it is so immensely comforting."

Kari Rose, who lives in Banks, Oregon, offers a nuanced perspective to the mental health and identity question of the person taking Trikafta. Growing up in CF Time, Kari experienced depression in her teens. "Being a teen is hard enough, let alone struggling with a terminal illness, and having these social gaps, and having to explain to people what is going on," she recollected. This mindset led to her not being as compliant with her treatments as she "led into this attitude of, well, I am going to die anyway." Kari never expected to have a family and decided not to get a degree because she anticipated dying in her thirties.

In February 2020, she began taking Trikafta. Her voice is "less raspy" because she is no longer coughing constantly, which allows her vocal cords to heal. Her PFT has gone from 43% to 71%. She now has a full-time job, and she is really wishing [she] had an accounting certification or a degree. However, contributing to society and her household income (with her husband) has given her a new way of understanding herself. She has new energy and new hobbies. Understanding this new life isn't simple though. Kari powerfully explains, "It is hard to be in our forties and fifties and have the health we wanted in our twenties." Instead of spending those years saving for retirement, she explains "Now we are so behind. We have the energy and drive, and now we have this new lease on life, but we are behind in the planning and the executing of all of that."

Kari also realizes how difficult it is to relate these experiences and sensations to family members and friends. "It is hard too for our families and close friends, and they see us with energy and as this new person; but we have to remind people we still have CF. We still have days where we do not feel well," she explained. She reflected that the days where those with CF are not doing well "can still be just as intense and hard; we just have fewer of them, and they are farther apart. It is confusing for those supporting us," she said.

I recognize it is hard to articulate these concepts to people who have not had these experiences. Although this is a fictitious example, one image to help explain the whiplash sensation of these Trikafta transformations is the original *Twilight Zone* episode "The Midnight Sun." This was the first *Twilight Zone* episode I saw as a child, and I was so moved by the twist that I sat agape, staring at the screen. The premise, established early in the narrative, is that the earth was moving closer to the sun and that soon most places on earth would be uninhabitable due to the extreme heat. Eventually, the entire planet would be so hot that life could not exist. Images of heat, melting paint, sweating, and dehydrated characters caused you to intuit the agony of the people and the increasing temperature. When the main character collapses from heat stroke at the end of the episode, viewers think this is the end and everyone will burn up. Instead, we witness snow blowing through a window and this same woman lying under blankets as her friend tries to keep her warm. The entire episode has been a hallucination. The earth is not moving closer to the sun, but farther away. The opposite of what we, the audience, held to be truth has been turned on its head. We learn that in two to three weeks there will be no life left on earth because everyone will *freeze* to death.

The young protagonist tells her elderly friend, as her fever begins to break, "Isn't it wonderful to have darkness, coolness . . . " And her friend, who fully comprehends the situation, wistfully sighs, "Yes, my dear, . . . it's . . . wonderful."[54]

The insights of Monique, Ben, Kari, and many others, bear resemblance to the total reversal of this story. They saw no reason, and no hope, to question the CF lens through which they lived their lives, just as viewers of "The Midnight Sun" had no reason to doubt the established story. Those moments when they realized that Trikafta really worked for them are pivot points that veered the trajectory of their life story in a different direction, from decline and death to improvement and life, just as the fictional story reversed from sweltering heat to bitter cold. In both cases, the reversal is extreme, unexpected, and doesn't remove all problems. It changes the parameters of the problems.

Many people taking Trikafta have experienced weight gain, resulting in a host of body image questions. Prior to Trikafta, I weighed around 140 pounds most of the time, as the mucus in my body blocked the absorption of nutrients and fat. When I would go in for my three-month checkup and get my weight taken before taking the breathing test, I would do everything I could to have my weight at about 145 pounds. Weighing in the mid-130s meant the PFT was down and IVs would follow. Weighing in the low 140s meant it was possible I would not have to do IVs, but there was still a chance. Therefore, I would eat a huge breakfast that morning and drink water before going to the appointment, trying to get every pound possible.

Most CF patients were told to eat as much as possible growing up because we would burn through calories so quickly. For many of us, we would never gain weight. At some point, I remember being told that 5,000 calories in a day should be my goal. Three to four meals a day, snacking between meals, adding desserts, and eating fast-food were all part of my CF diet. My friends were always

---

54. *The Twilight Zone*, "The Midnight Sun," directed by Anton Leader, November 1961.

envious that I could get multiple rounds at a buffet or not have to eat salads in my twenties and thirties. Weight gain was especially hard as I began running half-marathons. I would tell people I am running to clear my lungs, which made sense, and to gain weight, which left them confused. Given how much I ran, I needed to eat even more.

I remember the morning I realized I had gained weight post-Trikafta. I was getting dressed and I could not button my pants. My first thought was that the clothing had shrunk, so I grabbed another pair. Again, despite sucking in my stomach, I could not button my pants. Instead of being elated that I had gained weight after years of trying, I was deeply embarrassed. I didn't have a scale, so it was a few days before I weighed myself and saw that I was in the 160s. In that moment, I felt what many people experience when they feel ashamed about their weight. For me, it had the odd dimension of being both my goal and my source of shame.

It is impossible to explain the psychological and emotional change. I, and many others, went from being told to eat often and with no restrictions (all the while knowing you are fighting a losing battle and could never gain weight), to seeing you had gained 30 pounds or more. I had no idea that weight gain was part of Trikafta, which is partly my fault for not paying attention or researching the medication. I continued to eat large amounts of food for a month after I began Trikafta, before I had my early morning pants illumination. My immediate thought was, now I need to lose weight. I never had that sensation before.

Jess Pickering who lives in Connecticut, had similar thoughts on the weight gain aspect of being on Trikafta. She explained, "Weight gain is the big one. I weighed a lot less before starting it. . . . You go your whole life being told, 'You eat whatever you want.' . . . How do you change your life like that? You were conditioned to think 'I can eat whatever I want and not gain weight like everyone else.'" Like me, Jess is wrestling with the physical elements of the whiplash in diet and physical appearance. That doesn't mean Trikafta has been all bad for her. "I have an IRA, but if I didn't have Trikafta I wouldn't even bother," she explained. So, there are some aspects where Trikafta has been positive and has given her hope for her future. She explained that she no longer expects to be dead at age thirty-four. However, the physical changes and the difficulty of dealing with those changes are very real considerations too.

Emily Lawrence reflected on body image and weight gain as well.[55] "I was self-conscious about how skinny I was [before Trikafta]. . . . People talk about body shaming a lot, but not as often about being on the other end," she reflected. People always told her that she should eat more, but she was eating more food than her two older brothers. "Being a normal weight is weird," she confided. Like me, she had to throw out a bunch of her old clothes and buy a whole new wardrobe when she began taking Trikafta. "Sometimes I think, 'Man I feel fat,' which is weird because I never thought I would think that, . . . but my mom or fiancée will say, 'No, you are normal.'" It is hard for her to know what that means after going from being conscious about being too thin to gaining weight so quickly. It is like the whiplash effect from burning to freezing during "The Midnight Sun".

Weight was a huge part of the mental and emotional experience of going to the CF clinic every few months for my breathing test. The pre-Trikafta me would stare at a scale and hope to have numbers just a few pounds higher. At hospital visits, I would imagine myself as a rock thinking that would make the scale heavier. In a short time, the shame of my weight gain had me hoping for the opposite. I have had to change my diet greatly, which even includes eating an occasional salad! But the psychological issues remain because even when I was able to bring my weight to a more "normal" level by losing a few pounds, I still feel overweight. The quick change from being underweight, malnourished, and weak, to being a more appropriate weight, makes it impossible for me to gauge my healthy weight. Like wrestling with the mental health aspect of living longer, it is more about the change than the thing itself. It is great to be healthier and heavier, but it is outside of my realm of experience to know how to deal with these changes. Isn't it wonderful to be

---

55. Emily's Trikafta experience was described in chapter 5.

different from what I expected? I, too, can give the tepid reply, "Yes, . . . it's . . . wonderful."

One's identity can be attached to any number of things, and this loss of identity can be in areas outside of chronic illness. An occupation, an athletic achievement, or another person can become the central way a person sees themselves. Although I have never been a parent, I can imagine that having children grow up, leave the house, and begin a family, is a loss of identity for someone who has spent eighteen years (or more) identifying as a parent. Sure, one is still a parent, but the role of the parent as the sole caregiver shifts because children take on their own occupations, families, and interests.

As people age, their identity can shift based on losing their ability to do something considered important to them. My friend Nicole, who does not have CF, used to be a runner in college. She was very fast and enjoyed running. Now as an adult, she has very little time to run because of the demands of her job as a physician assistant. She recently told me how much she mourns this loss of her identity. When people ask her what she likes to do or how she spends her time, though she used to identify as a runner, she is unsure if that moniker still fits, or if she is a fraud saying this because she barely runs. Some people who have had such amazing experiences on Trikafta wonder if identifying as a person with a disability makes them a fraud as well. As Monique wondered, can she still be part of the CF online community when she does not have many of the symptoms of CF? What does it mean to have CF if you used to be horribly ill and now lead a seemingly "normal" life? Yes, it is a "good problem to have," but it is still an important question.

The questions presented in this chapter could form their own book. The mental health repercussions of Trikafta are some of the most powerful, fascinating, and confusing aspects of the Trikafta story. For those who have not had such an experience, this may make little sense. I know I am privileged. I know I am grateful. But I don't really know who "I" am. I just know that whoever this "I" is, he is not who "I" was before, and he is not the only one going through this experience. I am hopeful that sharing this experience will help me and others run a bit farther in the life race that was unexpectedly changed into a 26.2-mile marathon just as we were sprinting toward mile marker thirteen.

Transplanted Wisdom

The transplant community has been exploring the question of identity for years before gene modulators came along. Their insights into how to balance this can be helpful. Kassandra Klemenz had been in the hospital awaiting lungs for a few months with a lung function at 8% before a lung transplant saved her life.[56] She reflects, "Before my transplant, I [felt] like I was only identified as the sick person. . . . I took on that identity." Her friends and family viewed her as fragile, and she took on that persona. "I let peoples' judgment of me being that sick person [cause] me to take on that role," she explained. Following her transplant, she has been able to see that she is much more. Kassandra attends many athletic events that celebrate what her body can now achieve. When she is there, she does not introduce herself as someone with a lung transplant. "I don't feel like I am letting my organ donation consume everything about me," she explained. It is not that she wants to hide that she has a transplant. She wants people to see her as a conglomeration of many things: her talent, her hobbies, and her abilities. She stated, "I am so much more outside of this one thing."

Kassandra understands how people with Trikafta might be struggling with understanding who they are in light of all their life changes. "I feel like it's going to be an identity crisis for people. I felt like I had one," she recalled. Just as she identified as a sick person before the transplant, some people with CF take on this same designation. Trikafta could cause a similar identity crisis as she had after her transplant. However, she hopes that in the same way as her transplant allowed her to take on new ways of seeing herself, Trikafta will help those taking it to do the same. She reflected,

---

56. Kassandra's transplant experience was discussed in chapter 4.

"I hope they find . . . like myself, identities, and something other than the label of their disease." Kassandra, like Monique, has found a new identity not centered on illness.

Similar to Kassandra, Justin Goldsmith, sees a lot of similarities between the mindset of those on Trikafta and people who have had a lung transplant.[57] "I think a lot of what people who are doing well on Trikafta and people who are doing well after transplant [experience] is very similar," he explained. One of those similarities is the feeling of a "new lease on life." Justin's gratitude and new opportunities post-transplant are mirrored in the comments made by those on Trikafta. He empathizes with the struggles some are having with their mental health. Justin explained, "Struggling with your CF identity makes a lot of sense [when taking Trikafta]. . . . You are a new person in a lot of ways. . . . Now, having CF is in the back of your mind, whereas before it was in the front of your mind." While Justin acknowledges that his lung transplant maintenance is not something he can forget, there are aspects of having CF that are no longer his primary concern. Similarly, many people taking Trikafta describe forgetting they have CF at times when not long ago it was the central aspect of their identity.

Echoing Justin and Kassandra, Katherine Russell, understands the importance of shifting one's identity from being the sick person to something new.[58] She believes that her post-transplant experience of having CF "is not defining in most spaces" in the way that having CF used to be. One way she dealt with this transition was in her choice of a post-transplant career. "My work in the social justice space was kind of intentional, where the focus wouldn't be on my experience. It would be on someone else's. Rather than my identity focusing on the struggle of chronic illness, I began centering my identity on this thing that I am passionate about," she pointed out. Working for justice and reform in an area where others are experiencing injustice can shift the focus from inward to outward.

---

57. Justin's transplant experience was discussed in chapter 4.
58. Katherine's transplant experience was discussed in chapter 4.

Katherine created a new identity through her vocation of helping others who are suffering from marginalization.

Finally, Caleigh Haber also sees some similarities[59]: "I definitely see the connection. Whether someone has had a transplant or is on Trikafta, we're all navigating this unexpected extension of life that we hadn't necessarily planned for." Caleigh also made a connection to the way CF people see their bodies and how a transplant or gene modulator can change the way we see ourselves: "I think many of us can relate to feeling like we have a new body. A lot of people with CF struggle with body dysmorphia because we're so accustomed to being underweight and we think that is what looks good on us, and it is far from the truth." Having a transplant or taking a modulator that helps a person's body work more naturally causes a person to gain weight in ways they never thought possible. Caleigh explained, "Adjusting to the weight gain can be really difficult—seeing our reflection in the mirror, noticing the changes in our face shape, and how our bodies evolve. And this isn't something that only affects women; it's something men go through as well."

Caleigh offers a few important distinctions between transplants and gene modulators. Caleigh points out that a cure for CF would not mean the same thing to the lung transplant community because they have, in effect, traded one disease for another. They would still need to monitor for organ rejection and take countless medications. In terms of identity and mental health, Caleigh thinks that if she were taking Trikafta, she would see the possibilities for her future a bit more optimistically. "I still feel that my life is limited," she explained, pointing out that her life expectancy is still significantly shortened based on transplant survival statistics. "Those on Trikafta might share some of these feelings as well, but that is just my perspective," she mused. Many in the transplant community are more cautious than those taking Trikafta when thinking about the possibilities of a new lease on life.

---

59. Caleigh's transplant experience was discussed in chapter 4.

Those who have new organs have sat with the reality of a "new body" in ways that, while different physically, bear some similarity in understanding their identity. Those people need to be invited to the table where discussions of gene modulator identity are taking place. There are ways to have these discussions without conflating the procedures and risks these two groups face and, as Caleigh explained, without insinuating that the future prospects are the same. Many people in both groups can echo Justin's assertion that CF is being moved from the front burner to the back. Even if it is only for short periods, this relocation can cause one to have a seismic shift in how to view the person they see in the mirror. When you live every day, every moment of your life with a belief, and suddenly that core principle is relocated, disassociation is inevitable. This experience doesn't mean you aren't grateful and appreciative of the privilege of life. It means that you weren't prepared for the shimmering glare from the midnight sun.

Conclusion

Garden Privilege

The roses often tell their extravagant stories joyfully. Sometimes walking through the rose garden of life inspires people when they hear the roses speak. Those who have benefited from gene modulators, and some who describe their new lives post-transplant, can identify these changes as miracles. Unlike in fairy tales, however, miracles can have difficult side effects involving mental health and identity. When people articulate these struggles, they should be supported, not ridiculed for perceived ingratitude. Carrying a chronic illness may affect every aspect of a person's life and the way they understand Time, Space, and World. When a personal transformation and a shift of identity are added to an already difficult life, the results may appear unintelligible, even to some inside the same community.

Hilary Becker, who lives in Toronto, insightfully connected the elements of gratitude and privilege in the lives of those who have access to Trikafta. Hilary considered her condition to be "pretty moderate" until 2020, when she turned twenty-seven: "For about two and a half years, I was in the hospital dealing with persistent pneumonia, twenty-three kidney stones, pulling muscles in my back, . . . on IVs, doing homecare for months; . . . the ball was rolling in the wrong direction." She began taking Trikafta on January 7, 2022, which she described as "quite the saving grace." Things have reversed so much that her sweat test is now 26, which is below the threshold for having CF. "If I were to go into the hospital and get tested, . . . I would not be diagnosed with CF; it shows that my body is working right." Hilary realizes that these amazing effects would not continue if she lost access to Trikafta, which is a scary thought. She explained, "It is a unique experience to be alive and have your day-to-day well-being determined by [the] access that you have to a pill."

Hilary reflected on the wisdom she has learned from her CF experience:

> Why I'm doing it [treatments] is because I want to survive, and survival is a privilege that has been denied [to] so many people in our community. And survival may seem like the far end goal, but being able to do A, B, C, and D to get there, whether it is putting a needle in my thigh, or taking a pill, is a privilege. It may seem like, from an outside perspective, 'Oh that sucks that you have to do that,' but if I didn't, I wouldn't be alive. So, it is such a privilege to do those things. It's such a privilege to have Trikafta because other people don't.

Hilary is not minimizing the suffering of those with chronic diseases by saying they can get through things because it could always be worse. Rather, she is inviting those who have access to modern treatments, like Trikafta, to consider life without that access. It is not about comparing yourself to others to feel good that you are not them. It is about accepting the fact that those with access to treatments and medications would have worse CF manifestations without this access.

I echo Hilary's observation and find it to be great advice to myself when I begin to think how nice it would be to not have to use my therapy vest an hour a day, even with Trikafta. Hilary expressed that sometimes we wake up and feel like we don't want to do certain things, and it is a burden. Reframing that, she offered, "Imagine if you don't have any of that stuff, right?" Sure, I wish I didn't have to take Trikafta, but I am thankful every day that I can take it. . . . It doesn't suck for me to do it. It would suck NOT having it." That is the meaning of privilege. As we conclude the stories of transformation, hope, rebirth, and second chances, let us sit with the privilege of opportunity. Thank you, Hilary, for reminding me that "All these things are efforts to live, not burdens to carry." You can't hit the jackpot if you are unable to buy a ticket.

Part Three

Discarded Roses

In October 2023, I changed my health insurance provider. After three weeks I was told the new insurance company had twice denied the request to cover Trikafta. I began to worry and reduced my dose to a half-dose to increase how long the medication would remain in my body. By November, I had no more pills left to ration. My doctors and the *CF Foundation* continued to lobby for me to have access to the drug I had taken every day since January 1, 2020. Three days after my last dose, I began losing strength. I started coughing in the middle of the night, unable to sleep. By mid-November, I had lost around 10 pounds. I began journaling about the effects of being without Trikafta. The word that appeared most from this writing is "afraid." As a hospital chaplain, I was surrounded by illness and COVID-19 patients, yet I was without the medication that had kept me healthy. I wrote that going into the hospital each day was like "going into battle without a shield." My parents offered to find a way to pay the $25,000 it would cost to buy the medication for one month. I told them no. They had worked all their lives to save money for their retirement and I did not want them to spend it. I felt it would be unjust. I was scared and felt alone. I began looking for a new job and reached a conclusion: I would have to leave my program.

At the end of November, the insurance company relented and decided to cover the medication, perhaps because the re-enrollment period had passed, and they knew they would only have to cover it for one month. I still had to pay $1,500 for the month's supply but that was far less than the full cost. I had only written Part One of this book and had taken a break from writing. The day I resumed the medication, after being without it for nearly a month, I vowed to write until the book was finished. It was my wake-up call. I realized that access to Trikafta (or an equivalent) is an issue of justice that I had taken for granted. It was a reminder that there are many people for whom Part One is still their CF reality and Part Two is only their CF dream.

In the days after I resumed taking Trikafta, I began feeling ashamed that for nearly four years I had lived my life without being more aware of those in the CF community who were left out of the Trikafta revolution. While I know that "survivor's guilt" isn't always healthy or helpful, I came to realize that I did not appreciate the privilege of having Trikafta until I lost it. Mary Oliver tells us that the roses realize the heart-shackles are "lassitude, rue, vainglory, fear, anxiety, and selfishness." My lassitude, or lethargic inaction, arises from my selfishness and vain focus on my own well-being. Part Three will not only communicate why it is a moral imperative to continue CF research but also offer a glimpse into the lives of those on the margins of the CF community. Justice for these discarded roses and other people who do not have access to medical necessities is a moral imperative.

Chapter 7

Miraculous Letdown

My PFT dropped again. In fact, it dropped so much that the doctors think I need to do antibiotic treatments. Remember last year when I did them for the first time? I was so weak during the treatments and for weeks after I finished. I told the doctor that my martial arts team has been preparing for our national presentation for over a year, and we are going to compete at nationals. He said the longer I wait to do the treatments, the more the damage to my lungs could be long-term. It's just not fair. Why do I have to choose between my health and doing something important to me? Backing out now would crush my team and leave me feeling like I let them down. It seems like CF is constantly making me choose between my physical health and doing things that give me joy. What good is having physical health if I have to cancel important things with my friends? Goodnight.

Trikafta and other gene modulators have become revolutionary treatments for many people with CF. Some who have access to it and whose gene type indicates they would benefit have reported experiencing side effects that have ranged in scale from minor inconveniences to detrimental changes. I need to make it clear that I am not a medical doctor and that any decisions about taking or ceasing medication should be made in consultation with a medical professional. I am not making medical claims. I am reporting what some believe are side effects from taking Trikafta. Nearly 10 percent of those I interviewed reported some level of neurological changes. Some who described these issues were afraid to let me cite their name for fear that they would lose access to the medication, either through their CF clinic, insurance, or Vertex. I want to empower people to share their stories at least with their doctors, because only then will issues be researched and explored. I also hope those who have attacked or belittled people for sharing these experiences will realize the hurt that such accusations can cause. When the roses speak, we need to pay attention, even if their words are difficult to accept or understand.

Unmet Expectations

Laura Bonnell's experience as a CF parent led her to found *The Bonnell Foundation* in 2010. She explained, "The foundation is a support system for parents. We can relate because we are all going through the . . . same thing. *The Bonnell Foundation* gives financial assistance for CF-related medical needs and lung transplant grants." It also offers education scholarship grants for people who have CF. Laura continued, "We give grants to undergraduates attending a university, community college, or trade school."

Laura's two daughters, Molly and Emily, both have CF, and she was well aware of the progress in the early stages of gene modulator development. She recalls getting the message when Trikafta was approved in October 2019. She shared, "So as we are riding up the escalator from the basement of a conference, texts start popping up on my cell phone saying Trikafta was approved. I'm crying. I'm calling my husband . . .[and] my daughters. . . . No one is answering. I'm like, it's the biggest day and no one is answering!" Laura had waited for this day for a long time. It was a chance for her daughters to have access to a medication that could dramatically lengthen their lives.

Emily was sicker than Molly, so it was even more imperative for her to begin Trikafta. Laura reflected on those early days when Emily began taking it: "So, she goes on Trikafta and every day we are noticing, oh my gosh, you aren't coughing anymore. Your sinuses are draining." It was having a positive effect. After nine days, Emily told her mother about a rash spreading across her body. A short time later, she felt her throat starting to close up. Emily immediately went to the emergency room where they gave her an epinephrine shot. For the time being, she couldn't go back on Trikafta. Laura reflected, "So because it was our lifelong expectation that this was going to help us, we . . . were really depressed." The medication that was supposed to help Emily live longer had now become a danger to her life.

For the next two years, as her health worsened, Emily experienced issues with her mental health as she mourned the loss of the drug that had had such positive initial effects on her body. Laura confided that she had put pressure on Emily initially to get back on the medication, unknowingly making matters worse. At every CF appointment, she would try to convince her daughter to give Trikafta another try. Emily eventually expressed that she couldn't be pushed; she needed time. She needed to decide if it was worth the risk of experiencing side effects again. As Emily faced this decision, her mother tried to come to terms with a "miracle cure" that wasn't what she had hoped.

For two years, Laura tried not to pressure her daughter. Laura worried and felt powerless. Emily's health continued to decline. "Emily was getting sick, the worst I've ever seen her, with constant coughing attacks," Laura explained. But Emily is an adult, and it was up to her. Laura expressed that she was proud of how Emily coped with the situation. Emily reached out to an allergist to see if there was another alternative. Through a long process, doctors slowly reintroduced the medication into her body in liquid form over five weeks. She then began taking the medication in pill form. Almost immediately, she stopped coughing. The rash did not return. Both Emily and Molly can now take Trikafta and have experienced significant health improvements. Laura will never forget the two years when Emily couldn't take the CF modulator: "It's hard to watch your child go through something like this. You know there is a medicine out there that has helped [her], but it also harmed her until she could retry it. There is a lot of guilt to go around. I felt sad for Emily then, and I am so glad she's back on Trikafta. I can definitely sleep better. I also feel bad when I know there are many CF parents out there without their miracle drug yet, and that makes me sad and is something I think about daily."

Every medication can have the side effects listed on a package or distributed by the pharmacy. The rash that Emily experienced is described by Vertex as a possible reaction to Trikafta. Because each human body can react differently, anyone taking medication should monitor their symptoms and reactions closely and report issues to their doctor or pharmacist. Trikafta, as a newly approved medication, lists numerous potential side effects on the label. For example, in the introductory booklet sent to people with their first dose of Trikafta, several pages discuss the initial trials and the reported side effects. The headline reads, "Most common side effects experienced in a 24-week study in people taking Trikafta compared with those taking placebo." The most common side effects include headache (17%), upper respiratory tract infection (common cold) (16%), stomach pain (14%), diarrhea (13%), and rash (10%).[60] None of the side effects listed mention increased anxiety or other neurological issues.

While several people I spoke to discussed some of these physical side effects when they initially began taking it, most were able to navigate the physical symptoms long enough for those to wear off. In Emily's case, it took the ingenuity of an allergist who slowly reintroduced it into her system. Others have described psychological symptoms and how no one believed that these neurological changes could be connected to Trikafta. In 2022, an article in the *Journal of Cystic Fibrosis* entitled "Mental Status Changes During Elexacaftor/ Tezacaftor/Ivacaftor Therapy" explored the rarely discussed possibility of Trikafta influencing mental health. The article begins by acknowledging that CF-related mental health issues are not uncommon. The authors explain, "It is estimated 9–46% of people

---

60. Trikafta information published by Vertex Pharmaceuticals that comes with the medication.

with cystic fibrosis experience depression and 11–33% experience anxiety. This is comparable to or slightly higher than other complex chronic diseases of childhood."[61] The authors suggest that reduced quality of life, burden from treatments, medical costs, and other factors contribute to "symptoms of depression and anxiety."[62] Acknowledging the prevalence of anxiety and depression in the CF population, the authors studied six patients who began taking Trikafta and reported these symptoms. None of the six were taking medications commonly associated with altered mental status (AMS). The authors state, "To our knowledge, this is the first case series describing AMS in patients taking elexacaftor/tezacaftor/ivacaftor [Trikafta]."[63] In all six cases, the symptoms they noticed began within three months of being on Trikafta. The researchers also pointed out that "patients and CF care teams were unable to identify another plausible cause for these symptoms."[64] The following are words that those in the study used to describe their symptoms: fogginess, word-finding difficulty, less alert, memory issues, slurred speech, inability to comprehend reading, insomnia, dark/paranoid thoughts, and vertigo.[65] All six used the term "fogginess." In some cases, the patients, in consultation with their doctors, switched the morning and evening doses. The evening dose is one pill of ivacaftor, while the morning dose consists of two pills of elexacaftor, tezacaftor, and ivacaftor. Others took fewer doses to try to minimize these effects. The authors write, "In general, our patients expressed resistance to therapy discontinuation based on improvement of their lung function or other CF-related symptoms."[66] The authors surmise that underreporting of these types of issues may be due to patients fearing they will lose ac-

61. Suyeon Heo, David C. Young, Julie Safirstein, Brian Bourque, Martine Antell, Stefanie Diloreto, Shannon Rotolo, "Mental status changes during elexacaftor/tezacaftor/ivacaftor therapy," in *Journal of Cystic Fibrosis* (October 2021), 339.
62. Heo, *et al*, "Mental Status Changes," 339.
63. Heo, *et al*, "Mental Status Changes," 340.
64. Heo, *et al*, "Mental Status Changes," 340.
65. Heo, *et al*, "Mental Status Changes," 341–342.
66. Heo, *et al*, "Mental Status Changes," 343.

cess to the medicine, both during the trials and currently.[67] The authors conclude that there is no known medical reason for these reported side effects. They advocate for continued study and a "patient-centered approach to any modification of this therapy."[68] They state that "further research is needed to evaluate the specific impact of CFTR modulators on the central system."[69]

Some people described similar experiences to those cited in the study above from the *Journal of Cystic Fibrosis*. In some cases, these experiences have affected a person's life, but not to the extent of stopping Trikafta. One person who described his experience this way is Eric Verdon.[70] Eric wondered whether his experiences with anxiety stemmed more from Trikafta or the isolation of the pandemic: "When everything opened up [following the pandemic] having a simple conversation with somebody became a real struggle. . . . I get super nervous and sometimes sweaty, and this is not something I experienced in the past." For example, on his wedding day, he had more anxiety than he could have imagined, and these feelings often resurface over a year later. These heightened sensations have not caused him to stop taking Trikafta because the positives have outweighed the negatives. However, his search for the cause of his anxiety and his fear of talking to people, something he did not have before taking Trikafta, continues.

Others have had to modify their dose of Trikafta. Emma Boniface, thirty-five years old, lives in the UK and has had many of the same side effects from Trikafta mentioned in the study. In her teens and twenties, Emma was in the hospital every three months for IVs. By her late twenties, she took better care of herself, but her lungs had been scarred by all the years before. "I was still having quite regular treatment at the hospital just because of the neglect from years previous," she explained. Her PFT was in the low 30s when she got access to Symkevi (Symdeko), which brought up her

---

67. Heo, *et al*, "Mental Status Changes," 343.
68. Heo, *et al*, "Mental Status Changes," 343.
69. Heo, *et al*, "Mental Status Changes," 343.
70. Eric's consideration of having children was described in chapter 5.

lung function into the 40s. When she began Trikafta, she thought, "Oh wow, I am going to have this 20% or 30% increase and [instead] I think I got 8% and it just flattened out," she recollected. Trikafta did take away her CF cough within a few days though. She described this transformation as "mind-blowing."

Four months later, she began to have side effects. Emma explained, "And it was things like mood changes, [and] increased anxiety; but I didn't have anxiety pre-Trikafta. I wasn't on anxiety meds. . . . [After Trikafta], I was having issues remembering things and getting mind blanks." Emma had never had these issues before, and they began to interfere with things in her day that could be dangerous, "like leaving the hot tap on and the sink overflowing, or leaving the gas on after cooking dinner and then going into the kitchen two hours later, and . . . the gas is still on." Emma acknowledged that everyone forgets things from time to time, like where you put your keys or wallet. But this felt different. "My brain was . . . zapping out. [These things] were happening every day. And then it was weird because . . . I felt like I was in a thick fog, and I couldn't get my brain to compute. . . . So, remembering words [and] putting sentences together [was difficult]. . . . I couldn't focus on anything," she explained. Many of the symptoms Emma described were mentioned in the article, especially the idea of fogginess in thinking and reasoning.

Emma was having these issues before they were being talked about by the larger CF community. She brought these issues to her CF team. Thankfully, they believed her. "They were like . . . 'One hundred percent, we think it is happening; we have had other patients come forward and they described the . . . same thing,'" she explained. Other teams in the UK were not as open to this explanation. Emma reflected, "A lot of teams were like 'No, no. You know, it [has] nothing to do with Trikafta; it's all mental health'; or, 'You . . . have had such a shock that now your life is so different; it's just that you are adjusting.' . . . [and] a lot of people [are] being told, 'It's in your head; get on with it. Just crack on.'" Although her team could not provide an answer to what was going on, the fact that they believed her and did not just dismiss her experiences was so important for Emma.

Emma didn't want to stop Trikafta, so she and her team decided to give it six months. They thought perhaps in that time her body could adjust, and the symptoms would diminish. Unfortunately, "by month four I was just not able to cope, . . . to the point where I didn't feel safe driving. I didn't have the ability to put on the emergency brake. I didn't know if my brain would be able to do it," she confided. They decided to take her off the drug for a few months and reintroduce it at a lower dose. It was a difficult decision because she was the healthiest she had ever been. Emma went back on Symdeko and quickly became very sick. Emma describes, "It was horrendous. It was . . . three lots of IVs in two months. I was unstable. Cough and mucus, everything came back straightaway pretty much within the first week of being off it [Trikafta] completely." She decided she had to go back on Trikafta. Like some people in the study, she has reversed the morning and evening doses and takes two doses a week. The side effects are minimal, and her health is more stable. It is a middle ground where her body can tolerate the medication and it is doing some good. She works closely with her CF team as they try to figure out the best way to modify the medication.

Emma is glad that people are talking more freely about these issues now. She had numerous tests and has talked to other people who have had brain scans, to try to figure out the cause of the side effects. There are, so far, no answers. She explained, "In the UK, a lot more teams now are totally on side with it and say, 'Oh, we know it's doing it.'" This has been a welcome change in the past two years. Emma encourages people with CF to share their stories, especially in this time of new possibilities. Despite the setbacks of her Trikafta side effects, she sees a lot more hope for the future for people with CF. "I can talk about it because it is not all doom and gloom. . . . It's like a fairytale. . . . People should feel able to speak up and share their story," she encouraged. Emma's CF journey to Trikafta may not have come as easy as some fairytales, but she is grateful to still be alive to tell her story.

Like Emma, Beth Morgan also lives in the UK. She had a happy childhood growing up with CF. She reflected on how her physiotherapist [physical therapist] would come to her house with her sheepdog and she would do physical therapy on her while Beth did it on the dog. Reflecting on this memory made Beth smile. As she grew, however, the effects of CF worsened: "Into my teens, I was having IVs more regularly." She also did her best to hide her medical issues from people at school to not appear different from other teenagers. She stayed well enough to go to university and complete her degree; but by her late twenties, her decline hastened: "Into my thirties, I was having IVs every four to six weeks [and] a lot of exacerbations. I had to give up work, which is one of the hardest things."

In 2020, she began Kaftrio on a trial in the UK. "It made such a massive difference to my health, but unfortunately it came with a lot of side effects," she explained. After ten months, she had to stop the medication. Beth described "brain fog" and "fatigue" when taking it, as well as sound sensitivity: "I kept thinking the TV was really loud, but they [my parents] couldn't hear it." This also affected her mental health. "All I wanted to do was sit in the dark room and not speak. Music is such a big part of my life, but I couldn't listen to music for six months." She wondered if it would be better not to take it, and confessed, "So yeah, to really weigh your quality of life on it and your quality of life off of it. It presented a new problem. Part of me wished the tablet was never invented."

Beth no longer feels that way. After taking time off from Kaftrio, she decided to try again, in consultation with her CF team, this time at a low dose of two tablets a week. This cuts down on the lung exacerbations such that she is on IVs every five months, rather than every four to six weeks. The lower dose has decreased the horrible side effects as well. She reflected, "My attitude has changed a little bit because the low dose actually is helpful. . . . I am really grateful for it now." Beth indicated that her CF team was very supportive during her experience, and they never doubted that the side effects were real. She explained, "We looked at all the avenues. I went to get my eyes tested to make sure it wasn't my vision. I went to a neurology doctor to make sure it wasn't that, . . . [and] they were really willing to listen to me."

Beth desired to share what happened, so she posted a blog describing her experiences with Kaftrio. She got some online backlash for it. Though she didn't want to scare people from taking it, she wanted people to know that not every story was positive, that she had had huge expectations for the medication, and those expectations turned into disappointment. Like Emma, Beth must navigate the unmet expectations of a medication that has helped so many other people. Closely monitoring how it changes her body will be a continual aspect of her Kaftrio journey.

Kira, who currently lives in Florida, also experienced similar side effects to those documented in the *Journal of Cystic Fibrosis* study. Despite having stable lung function growing up, she reflects, "My doctors would pretty much from the age of nine say constantly, 'Oh, you won't make it till you are 18.' . . . It wasn't a very good thing to hear at such a young age." These comments contributed to her mental health challenges around her CF prognosis. Kira's form of CF has caused her more issues with digestion and sinuses, rather than her lungs. She has had numerous sinus surgeries and closely monitors her diet to avoid disrupting her digestive system.

Kira began taking Orkambi around the age of fourteen, eventually switching to Symdeko, and then to Trikafta. Trikafta increased her lung function, but before too long, she began noticing unpleasant side effects. "I developed really bad depression, which I hadn't had that bad for a long time." She informed her doctors and stayed on the medication, but the symptoms got worse. "I started having major vision issues," she explained. She has always had 20/20 vision, but she began seeing spots. "And it was bothering me because I saw spots everywhere. Especially when I was driving at night. I had to stop doing that." She began seeing eye doctors, who told her that everything was good with her eyes. She was told, "It is definitely the way your brain is perceiving things." Neurologically speaking, she also had trouble holding things. "I would have keys in my hand, and I would lose the grip," she recalled. Soon after that, she had occasional spasms in her legs and arms. None of these episodes had happened before taking Trikafta. Finally, similar to the cases in the *Journal of Cystic Fibrosis* study, she explained, "I started noticing that I would be talking to my mom or sister and I would say one thing, but then what I would be thinking was not what would come out."

Kira and her mother advocated for a lower dose of Trikafta, but initially, this was rejected. Kira recalls, "I don't want to be rude, but that is something that they never would consider." She expressed that it was impacting her mental health. "I didn't like that it was affecting me that badly." Her doctors eventually agreed to let her transition back to Symdeko. She waited a month for Trikafta to leave her system before changing treatments. "That whole month was not the best. I don't remember exactly. It was a little blurry, . . . and I was pretty jittery." Since she went back on Symdeko, the side effects have subsided, and her health has remained pretty stable. "I think in general, mental health-wise, it is a lot better," she concluded.

Kira's experiences with Trikafta and her mental health struggles mirror some of the side effects reported. Her comments that she could not form words when talking to her mom and sister sound similar to the study, as does her general sense of being less alert. Kira continues to battle with some of the CF problems associated with sinus and digestive issues but is grateful not to have the mental health struggles that she had during her nearly three years on Trikafta. Symdeko may not be as effective for some CF problems, but for now, she is happy to have it. Kira's Trikafta journey has been a difficult one. She confided, "I appreciate it. It is hard to get connected to other people with CF—the connection of knowing if someone understands even just a little bit [or] if they have had a similar journey with Trikafta." There are people out there who can help Kira know that she is not alone.

Eric has so far been able to weather the side effects, while Kira had to switch back to Symdeko. Emma and Beth find themselves in between, unable to receive a positive effect from Symdeko and struggling to find a dose of Trikafta that works effectively without side effects. In all their cases, Trikafta has not been what they imagined, nor what they perceived were the experiences of most people taking it. Sharing these negative experiences has sometimes been met with ridicule, causing them to feel even more alone. More people sharing their experiences will hopefully create an atmosphere of honesty and empathy. The full range of effects of Trikafta are still being explored. Whether it is a fairytale or a nightmare, each story must be heard.

Catch-22

Chronic diseases often present people with a difficult choice. When my uncle, Richard, was told he had an aggressive form of lung cancer, he was presented with options on how to proceed. One possibility was to take the more aggressive route of chemotherapy and radiation to kill the cancer, although this could leave him too weak to recover from the treatments. A second option was to go a less strenuous path, in the hope that it would be enough to slow the spread. He chose the aggressive approach. My father tells me that the pain he went through in the final months of his life, some resulting from the treatments trying to save him, was immense. In the end, neither approach would have made much difference because his cancer was in an advanced stage. He died less than a year after his diagnosis.

As a hospital chaplain, I was present at many discussions between families and patients on how to proceed with medical care. One powerful encounter I had was with a family I had accompanied for many months at the hospital. The patient, an elderly woman, had two code blues (her heart stopped, and CPR brought her back). She had been well enough to leave the hospital but found herself back on my floor a few weeks later, as her condition again deteriorated. Doctors wished to do a scope procedure to see if they could identify what was happening. The patient was very hesitant, perhaps fearing that if she was put to sleep, she might not wake up. Her husband agreed with the doctors that the scope was the only way to get more information. She asked me to offer a prayer for her uncertainty. Following the prayer, I attempted to normalize her fear without swaying her toward one decision or another. The next day they attempted the procedure, and her heart stopped again. Once again, they brought her back. Her body was now weaker than before. After a week, she was placed on CMO and died shortly after. Her heart gave out, worn down by the fight to survive. I did my best to comfort her family who supported her decision for her to have the scope procedure. In the end, if she was unable to survive the scope, she would not have been able to survive a more invasive procedure that would have been required. Like with my uncle, what appeared to be an important medical decision may not have made much difference in how long the patient had to live. However, similar to my uncle, this family had a moment where they had to choose, with potentially dire consequences.

Sometimes chronic illness decisions are not about life and death, but about quality of life in uncertain times. The opening journal entry was from my time as a college student, when I had to decide if I would do my treatments for three weeks and not be able to go to *Soo Bahk Do* martial arts nationals.[71] I had to weigh a year of training and preparation with my friends for a national event against doing what the doctors thought was best for my health. Such a decision does not have the weight of the previous two examples but is also very common within the chronically ill community. How does a person weigh the prognosis of a condition with the present enjoyment of being with loved ones? I suspect there are few people with a chronic illness who have never had to make this calculus.

Those featured in this chapter also have been faced with a difficult decision. One person who knows this well is Haley Moreland, who is twenty-eight years old and lives in Colorado. Like Kira, her CF manifestation was worse for her sinus and stomach issues than her lung complications. Her mid-twenties were very difficult: "My stomach issues, especially for a [woman] . . . feeling bloated all the time. It was just an awful experience." When Orkambi came out, she tried it but was only on it for a week when she had to stop because

71. Jimmy Menkhaus, "The Eternal Spring," in *With Every Breath*, ed. Katherine Russell (Merrill Press, 2006), 73–83.

of side effects with her stomach. "I wasn't digesting anything," Haley explained. When she was able, Haley started Symdeko. Her sinus and stomach issues continued to get worse.

In January 2020, Haley began Trikafta with the hope of having a gene modulator that worked with her system. She recalls her experience soon after starting it: "So I remember having a lot of stomach issues, I couldn't sleep, I had insomnia. Just a lot of stuff hit me. And I think the thing that I struggled with the most were the mental side effects." She attributed some of her experiences of fatigue and irritability to her insomnia. Soon, the fatigue turned into anger: "As it went on, I was very ragey, very, cagey. I couldn't figure it out because usually I am very logical. But if my boyfriend and I got into an argument, or [he] said something I didn't like, . . . and not just him, [but] anybody, . . . I was just looking to pick a fight. It didn't matter what you would say to me. You couldn't calm me down." Haley depicts a rage that was boiling within her that would get her upset at the slightest provocation. "Everybody was walking on eggshells around me." Over time, Haley's issues with anger decreased slightly and she became "overly emotional." "My depression and anxiety got so much worse," she explained.

After two years, she stopped taking Trikafta for a few months and currently has periods of being on and off of it, in consultation with her doctors. Some of the side effects remain, even over time being off the medication. "I completely changed. And [the anxiety] hasn't completely gone away. So, I don't know if those changes are permanent," Haley mused. She feels that if she wants to have biological kids, she will have to go on Trikafta again, and that scares her. "That is daunting, knowing I'll have to be back on it because I am overly sensitive. I think my relationships with people change when I'm on it." On one hand, she could take the medication and feel physically well enough to go out but be in such a bad mental space that she doesn't want to see people. Or, she could not take the medication and then not be physically well enough to go out. "[On Trikafta], I can go out with my friends, . . . run, live kind of a normal life, but mentally I don't want to. Is it worth it to be physically unable to do things (because you're fatigued, your lungs, your stomach, your sinuses) . . . or to be holed up inside [because mentally you are not up to it] when physically you can go out?" Would you rather be separated from the life you want to live and people you want to see because your mental health tells you it's not what you want or because your physical health tells you it isn't something you can do?

Haley doesn't want people to misunderstand how she feels about gene modulators and CF treatment advancement, even if it hasn't been great for her. "I don't want to come off like I hate the drug," she explained. "I have seen amazing stories with it [Trikafta]. I hope this is a step forward for gene modulators [and] for the future of CF patients," she offered with hope. For now, though, she is constantly reevaluating her approach and hoping that the next medication will work for her. Unlike Kira, who was able to go back to Symdeko, Haley's experience with previous modulators hasn't yielded success either. So, she waits and hopes. In the meantime, she weighs the no-win decision between her mental and physical health.

Haley's choice between her mental and physical health calls to mind the phrase catch-22, which comes from the novel, *Catch-22*, by Joseph Heller. The book, published in 1953, is set during World War II and explores the absurdity of war. In chapter five of the book, the author explains the concept of catch-22. If one was crazy, he would not have to fly the missions that were a risk to his life. But if he indicated he was crazy, by asking to not fly (a mission), he then demonstrated that he was not crazy because he was sane enough to ask. Thus, he would have to fly more missions. But he would be crazy to fly more missions. As Heller explains, "Orr would be crazy to fly more missions and sane if he didn't, but if he were sane he had to fly them. If he flew them he was crazy and didn't have to, but if he didn't want to he was sane and had to."[72] The catch-22 is a logical impossibility, a no-win situation. Haley wants to go out only if she doesn't take the medicine. If she takes the medicine, she doesn't want to go out.

---

72. Joseph Heller, *Catch-22* (Simon & Schuster, 1955), 55.

Jaime Dunaway also has experienced the catch-22 of Trikafta. She lives in New Hampshire with her husband and two children. Her first daughter was born in 2016, before Trikafta, and she had a difficult experience with the pregnancy. She explained, "I'm five feet tall. With pregnancy, the baby starts to press on your lungs, and you lose lung capacity. So, for me already having lower lung function and just being smaller in stature, there was significantly less area for the baby to expand into." She had a difficult time with her lungs at the end of the pregnancy, and she required a lot of rest and care once her first child was born. In July 2018, she began the Trikafta trial and could tell the changes right away. When she became pregnant with her second child, she had to leave the trial phase but was enrolled into regular access before her second child was born. Being on Trikafta helped during her second pregnancy. "From a CF standpoint, I did much better. And I was able to bounce back a lot easier," Jaime recalled. She had a 20–25% increase in lung function with Trikafta, which she described as "pretty great."

Unfortunately, Jaime had some significant side effects, some of which were similar to those in the aforementioned study. "I have had a lot of brain fog and trouble with my memory and pretty significant anxiety and depression. And issues like word-finding," she expressed. Jaime points out that these things happened during the trial, and she reported them, but there were so few examples that it was hard for doctors to say they had seen those side effects before. She currently takes only one of the morning pills. The symptoms have not completely gone away, but they have subsided. Jaime guesses she is getting "90% of the benefit" of a full dose. "So far, the benefits have managed to stay ahead of the negative side effects. . . . And to feel like I have to choose between my mental health and my lung health is a really hard place to be," Jaime concluded, echoing Haley.

Jaime continues to work through receiving criticism online and her own letdown. She is grateful that her doctors believed her when she reported what was happening. Unfortunately, some people have not been so supportive online. "A lot of it has come from parents who have kids with CF. There is a lot of, 'Well, my child has never had any problems,'" she explained. She clarified that she isn't trying to throw a "pity party." She just wants people to know that not everyone has had a great response to the medication. Some parents may respond harshly because they are afraid that the drug may be removed from the market if too many people report harmful side effects. One can see how parents, who have waited their whole life for their child to have a medication that may give them a chance at a more normal life would become especially defensive.

Jaime's own letdown is also difficult. Some people with CF follow drug trials closely and anticipate the possibility of a breakthrough. Naturally, this leads to hope for a better quality of life or even a longer life. Trikafta was hailed as the greatest breakthrough in CF research and, for those who have benefited from it, it has been just that. Jaime describes, "But I think having this . . . human desire to . . . place all your hope in this thing [Trikafta], that is going to be amazing and my life will be only great from here on out" can cause one to feel bad when it doesn't work out. Jaime has learned to deal with this by looking at her life and seeing other things that are important. Her challenge to herself is "to remember there is good in my life apart from Trikafta, with it and without it." She is now trying to be more attuned to seeing the small things in life, realizing that Trikafta is "not going to be my hope and savior."

Like Jaime, Andy Smith also has some concerns about Trikafta. Andy is thirty-eight years old and lives in the UK. Unlike many people I spoke to, Andy was sicker as a child than as an adult. He reflected, "I was really very poorly as a child. As an adult, I've actually been really healthy." He has not needed intravenous antibiotics for thirteen years, after having them every few months as a child. He spent his early life expecting to die before he was eighteen, and he described making choices as a teenager that reflected this expectation: "Because I thought, you know, if I'm going out, I'm going to go out with a smile on my face. . . . And then that nearly killed me." He began to turn his life around and got into fitness and living a healthier life.

When he began taking Kaftrio, Andy considered himself fairly healthy. He had an annoying unproductive cough, which Kaftrio took away within a few days of starting it. He also gained a bit of lung function, perhaps 5%. He is grateful for these positives concerning Kaftrio, but there have also been difficult side effects. One side effect that is listed on the medication is its impact on liver levels. Andy explained, "Very quickly I had to come off [one of the doses] because it was making my liver levels rise too quickly." It also began to affect his sleep schedule. He now takes Kaftrio in the afternoon, which has helped him sleep at night. Recalling Beth's comments about sounds, Andy became very reactive to noises: "Specifically around eating . . . I can't sit at a table with other people eating because the noise . . . gives me a really short fuse." He also suffered from mood swings, similar to Haley's "ragey" interactions with loved ones. All of these are symptoms he never had before taking Kaftrio.

Andy spoke of his Kaftrio experiences as a series of "pros and cons" and trying to make decisions based on those. "Because there's pros and cons to it," he explained, "and sometimes you have to . . . put up with the cons . . . because the pros are beneficial." For now, the pros outweigh the cons in his own experience. Andy is more concerned about the way people talk about Kaftrio than how it is affecting him: "My one issue is the lack of real-life experience that seems to get publicized about it. . . . Everything you see on social media is all, 'This is amazing!' . . . This isn't a wonder drug. And it actually comes with a few cons." He understands that adults can make those decisions for themselves. He is more concerned about children, who may not be able to voice to their parents what they are feeling while on the medication because they may not understand what is going on. He explained, "It's [approved] for children . . . between two and five years old that don't necessarily have a voice or opinion or experience; how are they going to deal with that?" He advocates for parents to be fully informed about the potential negatives so they can be aware, as much as possible, of what their children are experiencing. Andy concluded by stating, "I think sometimes people are too thankful for it, and they don't want to speak [badly] about it because other people are really positive toward it. We should be honest about it as a package."

During my time taking Trikafta, I have not experienced the extreme side effects described in this chapter. I certainly have not been brought to the brink of choosing between my mental and physical health. This does not mean I have not had mental health challenges in the past three years. After listening to the stories of those in this chapter and reading many others online while researching this book, I have wondered if my difficult mental health experiences were connected in any way to the medication. It is something that I monitor more closely now than at any other time in my life. I am grateful for those brave enough to share their experiences and want to encourage others to do so. Trikafta may act as a "cure" for some who have had their lives saved, but it is not a cure. The search for a true cure continues. The group that knows this well is the one whose gene type indicates that Trikafta would work, only to see their expectations unmet. For those caught in the catch-22 of their mental and physical health, Trikafta is either a "miraculous" letdown or a baby step toward what comes next. These roses need support, not guilt and shame, as they wait for the next step forward in their journey toward a longer and healthier life.

Chapter 8

The Collision of
Hope and Desperation

*There are a lot of times in my life that I have felt
forgotten. I am never picked first for anything in
class and am routinely overlooked by people I want
to date. Much of my life has been lived alone. I can
sit in a crowded room and know that I am different. Perhaps this is something I have carried over
from my time in college. As an adult, it isn't much
different. CF can make someone feel like no one
in the world knows the true me. Goodnight.*

If the roses of chapter 7 exemplify the word "unheard" as they
have tried to communicate their experiences with Trikafta, those
in chapter 8 might be described as "abandoned." While chapter 7 is
about those whose gene type indicates that Trikafta should work,
chapter 8 is about the opposite. For these roses, their gene type,
known as "nonsense mutations," does not benefit from the current
gene modulators. While the research continues for an equivalent,
it is made more difficult by the numerous mutations found within
this group. Not all nonsense mutations are the same, complicating
the search for a way to treat them.

The whole CF community was previously united in their search
for a cure. With many now benefiting from Trikafta, the loud shout
from the base has become a light whisper from the margins. People
who stood shoulder to shoulder have now been separated, as many
who have been "cured" can run ahead and experience life, leaving

the 10 percent to wonder when their opportunity will come. While it can be hard to see this happen, it is even harder when the research slows and resources get diverted away from CF research, especially as the common CF narrative talks more about Trikafta as a cure, rather than Trikafta as an innovative step. Listening to these roses share their feelings of abandonment and pain is a reminder that there is more work to be done. It is a moral imperative to not leave a job unfinished. Even if many in the CF community have been changed by gene modulators, it is an injustice to neglect others as they fight for the same chance at life.

Fractured Community

One member of the 10 percent is Sarah Skeffington, who lives in Columbus, Ohio with her husband Joe. Sarah recently turned forty, a milestone for those with CF. There were certainly times in Sarah's life when she didn't expect to make it to forty. Sarah grew up in Sacramento, in a very supportive community. She remembers going to "hospital camp" and interacting with other people with CF: "We also had cancer patients and transplant patients [at the camp] and you were in hospital rooms with other people. I think the social aspect of the disease was so critical to my own awareness and how I accepted it." As a young child, having people around her who also faced unique challenges helped Sarah process her identity. She continued, "I loved CF camp. I loved being with people like me. I think that was so healthy. And, of course, we all got pseudomonas together one year because someone had pseudomonas . . . so I have had that since I was eight."[73] Sarah doesn't speak with regret or anger about getting pseudomonas. Rather, she speaks with gratitude about how the camp helped her to know she was not alone.

---

73. Pseudomonas is a common pathogen in the lungs of people with CF. It can be difficult to treat and can cause further progression in the disease and a decline in lung function over time. It can also cause infection and inflammation.

Sarah's CF life began to change when her family moved to Delaware when she was twelve. She left the supportive community she had known and moved to a place where having CF caused her to feel singled out: "And so, [in] my first class, I remember being super self-conscious and uncomfortable. And that was really the first time in my life that I felt that way about my CF." Cross contamination rules also began around that time, limiting her ability to have contact with those struggling with similar issues. Sarah reflected that during a hospital stay where she had been initially with another person with CF, twenty-four hours later they were separated: "I remember the hospital . . . going into lockdown, and the hospital staff were like, 'Oh, no. You're not supposed to be around other people with CF,' and I was like 'Excuse me; since when? We have all grown up together. Are you telling me I can't be around people like me?'" It is a powerful way to realize that you are different from other people and can't even find comfort among those like you.

In 2007, Sarah moved to Texas to live with her aunt and uncle and faced even more challenges. When her father's job changed six months later, she lost her health insurance: "They missed somewhere in the paperwork, and they didn't pick me up and they couldn't get me back. So, completely uninsured . . . I was without insurance for probably a year. I lost 70% of my lung function and 25 pounds." Sarah had a job that did not offer health insurance, and she did not have the money to pay for it. "I have been fighting an uphill battle ever since," she said emotionally. One hospital was willing to treat her, but only for three days: "I remember sitting in that doctor's office and the doctor telling me 'You don't have insurance. That is a death sentence.' And I was just sobbing. I was angry and crying, mostly because I was angry. I was born with this. I didn't wake up one morning thinking, you know what, this would be a really great idea to have a chronic illness where I would need health insurance for the rest of my life." It was the sickest Sarah had ever been, and the response was not one of empathy, but blame for not being able to afford the care she desperately needed fighting in CF Space.

Sarah got married in 2009 and has regained some of the ground she lost during her experience in Texas. The CF infections over the years have certainly taken a toll on her body. She explained, "My pseudomonas and my MRSA are to a point where they are very hard to treat because I'm resistant to everything. I'm still very active. For six years I slept [using] oxygen." Sarah continues to do all she can for her body to fight off disease without resorting to medications, as her body becomes resistant.

Physical trials are not the only ones Sarah faces. There are also social and emotional valleys within the CF community. Harkening back to when she was removed from the room of another person with CF, Sarah describes the fracturing of the CF community. This is the difference between her, as a member of the 10 percent, and others who have CF. Prior to Trikafta, Sarah was very connected to people with CF through online communities, gaining strength and inspiration from hearing about the ways others tried to remain healthy. For example, comparing run times and setting half-marathon goals helped her feel she was not alone in her battle. Sarah emotionally reflected,

> And almost in an instant, the tight-knit groups of active CF'ers . . . were gone—just vanished, like we didn't exist, never part of the same club. It was almost jarring, how quickly it evaporated. All of a sudden, all of these people [who] were in the same boat as you are no longer in the boat, and you're still in the boat. They got the life raft and you're sinking. That was probably the first time in my life I really questioned, why me? Why didn't I get Delta 508? Why did my cousin get Delta 508 and not me? Probably the first time I have ever felt selfish about my CF. And a little bit angry I wasn't part of that group. You just stopped hearing from people; you stopped hearing about their outdoor adventures because they were healthy. They got to live their lives.

In the past few years, Sarah has worked to process these emotions and feels she is in a better place. She still feels the anger and abandonment from time to time but has been able to reframe it: "It's probably taken a couple of years to level out my mental experience with not feeling like it's hopeless but also balancing that hope with reality. Chances are I'm not going to see anything like Trikafta for me in my lifetime." Sarah continues to work on how to exist with this dichotomy, a daunting task for someone also trying to navigate a fractured community, while everyone else on the sinking boat has safely made it to shore.

Jarrod Landau is also a member of the 10 percent. He currently lives with his family in Australia, after previously living in Spain and Israel. Other than doing his treatments for two hours each day, CF didn't affect his childhood. When he moved from the children's hospital to the adult clinic, his prognosis with CF was explained to him by one of the doctors. Jarrod recalled, "The doctor said to me, 'Look, the lungs aren't that great. You will probably need to get a lung transplant at twenty-seven.' So, that was news to me." That conversation brought Jarrod to the realization of what it means to live in CF Time.

At twenty-one years old, Jarrod decided to be more health conscious. He stopped drinking and began going to the gym regularly. Although his lung function is currently down to around 40%, he feels pretty good, and at fifty, he is grateful to be as healthy as he is. The slow decline, rather than extreme lung function loss, helps him to keep active. Jarrod offered, "I think the lungs really allow you, as long as you've got a slow decline, [to not feel it] as much as with the sharp declines." Jarrod also credits having a positive attitude: "I think the disease suits my personality to be honest, because I am able to handle it."

As a member of the 10 percent, Jarrod has the added component of not only fighting CF but being left outside of the current gene modulator treatments. Jarrod shared, "Although I feel I'm jealous, [because] you know, of course, we all want something where I don't have to worry about my lung health again; that would be amazing. But I don't know, maybe something better will come along in the next few years, something to really catapult everyone in the community, not just the people in the 10 percent." Until then, Jarrod does all he can to stay active and healthy, spending time with his family and working as a foreign exchange trader. His hope for something to help his health in the future is balanced by his appreciation for what he has in the present.

Jarrod is inspired by all that Emily Kramer-Golinkoff has accomplished for the 10 percent: "Emily is amazing—incredible! You can do your medicine, you can do exercise, you can have a positive attitude, but unless you try to work to better the long-term, like Emily is on health or research, you . . . are missing a piece of the pie. So, I try to do as much as I can with her." Emily's nonprofit, *Emily's Entourage*, is doing just what Jarrod described. She is leading the way for research for the 10 percent, making sure that, in an era of fractured community, the 10 percent are not forgotten.

Emily was diagnosed at six weeks old. No one in her family had CF and it hit her parents hard: "It came as a huge shock. I was their first child." Emily had her first hospitalization when she was in the fourth grade and missed a lot of school in the seventh and eighth grades. She recollected, "It was the first time I was ever really scared with CF." Adhering to treatments in high school enabled her to remain relatively healthy. College was a different story: "I really struggled. I spent most of freshman and sophomore year on IVs. I . . . struggled to juggle everything. I burned the candle at both ends." Emily described similar issues as others when meeting new people in college. Navigating who to tell and how much to reveal about yourself is a daunting task in a new environment. Eventually, Emily adapted. The year she graduated from college, 2008, is also the year she was diagnosed with CF-related diabetes: "I lost a significant amount of lung function and I was never able to recover." Since that time, she has been living with a lung function in the 30s.

Despite living with a deteriorating lung function, Emily co-founded *Emily's Entourage*, in 2011, to speed up the development of lifesaving treatments and a cure for those in the final 10 percent of the CF community who do not benefit from current CFTR modulators. Emily explained, "And the reason for starting [it] is we saw that the CFTR modulators were coming down the pike. That was right before Kalydeco. We saw the scientific community quickly turning all their attention to Fdel508." Emily understands why, given the prevalence of that mutation in the CF community. Those with non-Fdel508 mutations, including nonsense mutations and other rare mutations, knew that the research trajectory would not offer them the same results. Emily continued, "Not only was there nothing imminently coming, but there was no infrastructure to develop those sorts of things in the future, and nobody was paying attention to it in a coordinated, strategic way. It really came from the collision of hope and desperation." It is from this urgent need for leadership and coordination that *Emily's Entourage* was born. Emily knows that she and others in the 10 percent are living on borrowed time.

The organization focuses on "accelerating research and drug development for those who don't benefit from existing therapies and [is] trying to make things happen fast because time equals lives." To meet this goal, they have given out thirty-eight research grants around the world and "have a venture philanthropy arm where [they] give out strategic investments to companies developing therapies." They also have a patient database and clinical trial matchmaking program to help speed up trial recruitment and connect people to potential trials. This is helpful because they go directly to the patient community, rather than going through hospitals, to make connections for the trials. They also have a major fundraising gala each year and other annual campaigns. *Emily's Entourage* is actively moving the research forward in search of new therapies.

Emily expressed that she is happy for the way Trikafta has changed the lives of those who can access and tolerate it: "We're so thrilled. Some people describe it as bittersweet, which has never felt accurate to me because there is nothing that feels bitter about it. . . . It is just that we . . . want it too, and time marches on, and our disease marches on." It is the left behind aspect of the fractured community that Emily said causes fear and sadness in the 10 percent community: "A lot of people feel incredibly left behind; a lot of people feel . . . scared that the scientific community is going to turn away [and stop doing CF research]. . . . People feel very isolated." These are the feelings that propel Emily's work forward, fighting for those who feel they are placed on the outside or, as Sarah described, those who did not get on the life raft. The fragmentation of the community has also left fewer resources for those who battle the disease without gene modulators. Emily described how it is harder to attract companies to work on therapies because the number of those who would benefit is smaller. She shared emotionally, "It's a small portion of the community now that is bearing a disproportionate amount of the weight."

Emily explained that even the notion of "10 percent" is misleading. She elucidated, "We say the final 10 percent, but it is fairly inaccurate because it is so much bigger than that." She mentioned those who can't tolerate Trikafta and the people who do not have access to it. In some countries, many people do not even have access to technology to assess if they have CF or modulator-eligible mutations. When seen this way, it is not a battle for the "final 10 percent." It remains a battle for the CF community, a battle that Emily will continue to advocate for as long as she is able. Although Trikafta has split the CF community, Emily reminds us that we are all the same because we are all holding out for a cure. In the future, everyone in the CF community will benefit because Emily did not give up her fight at the intersection of hope and desperation.

The Search Party

Will Corcoran is a member of the 10 percent. He had a liver transplant at the age of fifteen, an uncommon CF occurrence. As he grew older, his lungs became the primary concern. Will described his current treatment regimen: "I nowadays do four breathing treatments a day, sitting at my desk for two hours each day, minimum." In the past few years, Will has had to cycle between IVs and oral antibiotics, with only a few weeks off from medication between cycles. This increased usage has made him resistant to some of the medications. Doctors continue to cycle them, but there is only so much they can do.

Will describe his feelings about Trikafta by reframing them in a helpful way: "I haven't benefited from a modulator, but when Pulmozyme came out, I was six or seven, and I would think that people who were . . . my age back then were in a similar type of situation . . . I have benefited from a lot of amazing drugs." He also values his role as a mentor for younger folks with CF, many of whom are benefiting from Trikafta. "I know my time will come," Will offered, optimistically. As a person with cystic fibrosis, he feels privileged to live in the United States because if he lived in many other countries, he would not have access to his level of needed CF care.

Just like Emily, Will thoughtfully articulated the need for expediency given his decline: "I am not going to be able to battle CF [in this way] my entire life; it is not sustainable. I can still die at a very young age because the medications available to me right now are not enough." This is especially complicated by his increased drug resistance. Once the current drugs no longer work for him, he will be out of options. Will explained, "For people like me, there is going to come a time [when] I have to choose to get a lung transplant, [which] basically forgoes the opportunity to be on a highly effective modulating or gene editing [medication]. And if I do that, there is no going back."

Will brought up an important aspect of the final 10 percent. He explained, "Among the 10 percent there is a higher incidence of these people being people of color. Among the 10 percent of people not on modulators, that community is made up of 40 percent people of color, [whereas] among the entire CF population, it's less than 5 percent." In describing this demographic, he referenced the historical experiences of people of color in the US and their mistreatment by the medical community. "That is all the more reason why you can't leave [them] behind," Will implored.

One of the important themes of my work as a chaplain was coming to terms with the history that Will mentioned, about the way people of color have been minimized or ignored by the medical community in the United States, and how chaplains play a role in making sure all patients' voices are heard. To put the injustices of the health care system into context, one needs to listen to and learn from the voices of people of color who tell about their history in the US. During my residency, I read *White Rage*, by Carol Anderson.[74] Anderson's methodical exploration of US history, through the lens of the Black community, demonstrates to me the cyclical nature of racism, which appears differently in each generation. A central message of her book is the reaffirmation of the subjugation of the Black community through rules and laws of discrimination.

Having a deeper understanding of the history of discrimination led me to see how this history connected to healthcare and why some people of color may not trust medical professionals. The quintessential example of racism in healthcare is the Tuskegee Syphilis Study, from 1932 to 1972, which involved 400 Black men. The participants in the study did not give consent and were not treated, even when treatment was available. More than 100 people died from the "experiment" of observing the effects of the disease when it is untreated. In her essay, "Under the Shadow of Tuskegee: African Americans and Healthcare," Vanessa Northington Gamble explains why this atrocity needs to be seen in the wider context of the Black experience of American healthcare. She writes, "For many Black people, it has come to represent the racism that pervades American institutions and the disdain in which Black lives are held. But despite its significance, it cannot be the only prism we use to examine the relationship of African Americans with the medical and public health communities."[75] The abandonment of the 10 percent, which contains a high percentage of the CF community's people of color, is another example in this long arc of medical racial disparity.

---

74. Other books we discussed in residency were Resmass Menakem, *My Grand-mother's Hands: Racialized Trauma and the Pathway to Mending Our Hearts and Bodies* (Central Recovery Press, 2017), Mary-Frances Winters, *Black Fatigue: How Racism Erodes the Mind, Body, and Spirit* (Berrett-Koehler Publishers, 2020), and Robin Diangelo, *White Fragility: Why It's so Hard for White People to Talk about Racism* (Beacon Press, 2020).
75. Vanessa Northington Gamble, "Under the Shadow of Tuskegee: African Americans and Healthcare," in *American Journal of Public Health* vol. 87, no 11 (November 1997) 1777.

During a chaplain visit, I sat with a young woman of color who expressed anger about her treatment at a nursing home. She had cancer and came to the hospital quite often for treatment. She felt that those at the nursing home were not listening to her when she told them she needed to be taken to the hospital. Her frustration led to tears. Referring to the other residents who were much older and sicker, she exclaimed emphatically, "If they don't listen to me, a person who can speak, how can we expect them to listen to people who can't speak," I encouraged her to continue to speak her truth. As she spoke, I thought of *White Rage* and the way people of color have been marginalized in our society. I left the visit feeling shame for her predicament while being inspired by her tenacity. In my studies as a chaplain, I became more attuned to the ways people of color are ignored. The lack of support for the final 10 percent isn't an outlier in this story. It is an indicator of an ongoing narrative.

Like Will, Steph Hansen is also a member of the 10 percent. She is in her mid-thirties and lives in Texas. Until the age of thirteen, her hospitalizations were infrequent. By her early twenties, she began to decline: "In my early twenties, I was getting admitted every other month or so. It was exhausting." She tried to slow this descent by getting into fitness and being more compliant with her treatments. Given her number of hospitalizations, her system developed allergies to the medications. Her CF team only admits her when she is so sick that she is in a lifesaving situation. Her doctors have told her, "To expose your system to these antibiotics, we are taking a huge risk every time." When she is admitted for IVs, she begins treatment in the ICU. This is to try to figure out which medications will affect her bacteria. "It has become really intense and scary," Steph described emotionally.

As Steph's condition has declined, she has watched many in the CF community improve: "It's been a tough few years, living in that margin of people who can't take Trikafta . . . and I've watched the community take off." Through her emotional and physical pain, Steph fought to hold back tears as she described how she is running out of time. She shared some of her emotions around getting closer to her death and hoping something will come along that can help her live a bit longer. "I have really intense feelings about being forgotten and left behind," she offered in vulnerability. She is happy for those in the community who benefit from Trikafta. Like everyone in the 10 percent, she wants the same opportunity for life. She admitted, "But I can't deny the part of me that's so desperate and feels so powerless." Steph was in an online chat with other people in the 10 percent and they were asked what emotions they felt. Nearly everyone said, "bittersweet." When it came to her, she said in honesty, "I feel desperate." She wonders if she was the only one feeling that way, or if other people did not want to share their real emotions. That experience "sort of added to the isolation that I felt around my emotions, so that has been an interesting part of the experience," she explained.

Steph comes from a military family, which informs how she sees the way the 10 percent have been treated. When people ask her why it is important to continue to work for the final 10 percent, Steph says emotionally, "I'm like, are you kidding me? . . . When a person goes missing in war or they get captured, . . . the response is to go find that person; the resources spent on one single person to try to find them—we will sacrifice other lives. . . . Why are you asking me if my life is important?" Steph explained how frustrating it can be to have to explain why her life is important. She tearfully concluded, "That's why my life is important. Because every life is important."

Steph continues her advocacy for CF research whenever she is well enough. She knows the clock is counting down and each time she gets sick, she may not be able to recover. From a young age, she has lived in CF Time while remaining hopeful and passionate about the possibility of a cure. She watches the second hand of the clock move around faster, baring the scars of each battle, as she fights to hold on to the ground she is losing. Battling CF, while also battling the notion of being forgotten, makes the fight doubly difficult.

Steph's insight about the way people will spend time and money to rescue a soldier in the field called to my mind two examples in recent memory. First, the publicity of the Tham Luang cave rescue of the Thai football (soccer) team, in the summer of 2018. The team and their coach were trapped for three weeks, a story that captured the hearts of people around the world. All the boys and their coach were successfully rescued. Rescue efforts involved more than ten thousand people and cost perhaps $500,000.[76] Even more recently, the failed rescue attempt of the wealthy tourists who died going to see the Titanic on the submersible cost the government at least $1.2 million. In this case, the tourists chose to go into danger, knowing what could happen. The rescue effort captured the attention of the world, as people waited each day to see if the rescue would be successful. Steph is right. These lives are important; her life is important because every life is important.

While the philosophical argument for continuing to work for treatments for the 10 percent is strong, a mathematical argument can also be made. When one hears the difference between 90 percent and 10 percent, it may be tempting to think that is a large number. Reframing those numbers can be incredibly helpful. According to the *CF Foundation*, in the United States, 40,000 of the 341 million people have CF (.012%). The same source estimates that approximately 105,000 of the nearly 8 billion people in the world have CF (.0013%). Apparently, many people feel that searching for a cure that affects .012% of the US population and .0013% of the world population is a good use of resources, as evidenced by the huge amount of time and funds dedicated to CF research. If it were merely about numbers, one could argue that *no* research into finding a cure for CF makes sense. Those percentages are a very small number of people. Those who think that research should stop because "only" 10 percent of the population can't use a modulator argue that there is a statistically meaningful difference between .012% and .0012% in the US and .0013% and .00013% globally. It is morally incongruent and mathematically inconsistent to hold this point of view. It is time to break the cycle of history that regards people of color as less worthy of equal care. On this rescue mission,

76. Jye Sawtell-Rickson "Quantifying the Thai Cave Rescue," *Medium*. September 28, 2018. https://jyesr.medium.com/the-thai-cave-rescue-248c5b-08cbf0.

everyone needs to be brought home; they can't hold their breath much longer. For it is only in saving everyone that we can truly save ourselves and lift those who are sinking on the corner of hope and desperation.

Chapter 9

Born Under
a Different Star

Today we visited a sick boy in a remote Honduran town. He was lying on blankets with his body twisted like a question mark. He seemed unable to communicate and barely aware of those around him. On our ride back to town we were told that he did not have much time to live. Although he did not have cystic fibrosis, as I sat next to him, I reflected that if I had been born in many other countries, I would not have survived infancy. I was lucky. This boy was not. Access to lifesaving medication is not only dependent on the time one is born but also equally dependent on the place. I don't think I will ever forget him. Goodnight.

Access to modernized healthcare varies around the world. More affluent countries often have access to equipment and medications that are nonexistent in more impoverished areas. Treatments for cystic fibrosis follow a similar path. Access to enzymes, nebulizers, and therapy vests have always been sought by people who live in countries where these are scarce. The existence of gene modulators has served to exacerbate the difference between those who have access to these medications and those who do not because these treatments are often so effective. The cost of Trikafta, approximately $25,000 per month, coupled with the miraculous effects of the medication have caused increased pressure on government entities, insurance companies, and Vertex Pharmaceuticals to make these medications accessible. Even the most affluent person would struggle to pay for Trikafta out-of-pocket, so financial assistance is necessary in some form. While there is no easy answer for how to make access to gene modulators more prevalent, it is imperative that progress is made as soon as possible to get these medications to those who need them.

Successful Advocacy

During July 2021, I participated in a thirty-day silent retreat at Eastern Point Retreat Center in Gloucester, Massachusetts. During the pre-retreat orientation, I mentioned that I felt drawn to spend thirty days in silence to reflect on how to spend my "bonus years" that I never expected to have prior to Trikafta. On the first break day, ten days into the retreat, when talking is permitted, I was approached by one of the retreatants, named Suzy McCall. Suzy is a missionary living in Honduras. She mentioned that one of the high school students she works with, named Andrea, has CF. She wondered if it would be possible to get her this "miraculous" medication. She requested the name of it and said she would make a few phone calls. That evening, as we were preparing to go into silence for ten more days, Suzy found me in the library. Her face appeared downcast. "I made some phone calls. . . . There is no way we can pay for that drug. It's too bad. She isn't doing well."

For the rest of the retreat, whenever I took Trikafta I thought of this young girl that I will never meet. A few times, I stared at the pills before ingesting them, contemplating how I was alive because of a small tablet. I asked myself why I was lucky enough to be born in a place that had access to modern medical treatments and wondered why I get to live a bit longer than those who can't get Trikafta. I felt a sense of survivor's guilt, and I can only guess this is how it might feel to be in an accident where one person walks away without a scratch and the other is taken to a hospital in critical condition.

Candace Taylor worries about her daughter Isla having access to Trikafta when she is old enough to take it. Candace knew little about CF before her daughter tested positive after her birth, and she remembers little about the phone call with the geneticist. "I couldn't tell you a lot of what was said because it was so shocking," she recalled. Isla is now fifteen months old. Her primary CF manifestations have not been her lungs, but her digestive system. While things are currently under control, it can be difficult for Candace to face Isla's future without some sense of trepidation: "When they first told us her diagnosis, they said, 'You know, it isn't a death sentence anymore.'" The doctors especially highlighted gene modulators like Trikafta. Candace continued, "Then they drop the price tag. . . . That is five times my wage." There are programs that can assist with the cost in Canada if neither Candace nor her husband has a job with benefits, but it is still a scary proposition. "There are a lot of hoops to jump through," Candace explained. And there is always the uncertainty of accessibility when Isla is old enough to take it. Candace's fear of the possibility of not being able to get access to a drug that could greatly help her daughter was apparent in her voice: "Just because it is a rare disease doesn't mean it should be a rare drug."

Trikafta is accessible in Canada because of people like Beth Vanstone. Beth's daughter Madi was diagnosed with CF shortly after birth. She was very sick growing up with sinus, stomach, and lung issues from CF. When the opportunity arose for a study for Kalydeco, Beth enrolled her eleven-year-old daughter. "I didn't even have an understanding of what it was," she confessed. However, doing anything she could that might help her daughter was paramount. Within two days of starting, Madi told her mom, "Mommy, I can breathe through my nose." Her transformation brought up her lung function from the 50s to 115%. "It was miraculous," explained Beth, "until this trial was over and she [no longer had] access."

Beth and Madi began to lobby parliament for access to the gene modulator. "I strongly felt they couldn't let an eleven-year-old die," Beth explained. Their efforts garnered the attention of various news outlets in Canada as they lobbied to save Madi's health. They held press conferences, gave interviews, and attended CF advocacy days. After a two-year battle, Kalydeco was approved for funding, in 2012.[77] Their advocacy for public funding for the first CF gene modulator was a success that saved many lives.

Madi switched from Kalydeco to Trikafta once it became available in Canada. "Having Kalydeco made a huge change. Having Trikafta has taken it to another level," Beth explained. Before starting Trikafta, Madi's PFT had fallen back into the 80s but is now back above 100%. As for Madi, she can pursue her love of photography and has a chance at a life that, without gene modulators, she and her mother never dreamed possible. For a mother who would do anything to help her daughter, it is a relief that her work was a success: "It just feels like a huge weight has been lifted off my shoulders." The advocacy Beth and Madi did for access to Kalydeco paved the way for access to the gene modulators that followed. They are an example that sometimes working hard for what is right can bring about lifesaving success.

Jess Ragusa also has firsthand experience advocating to bring Trikafta to a country.[78] In 2020, she was unable to meet the threshold to get Trikafta on compassionate use grounds, and the Australian government was unwilling to subsidize it. In 2021, she began coughing up so much blood that she and her family decided to do whatever was needed to get access to the medication. She explained, "My family remortgaged the house so we could start to pay privately for Trikafta. It was costing us 21,000 Australian dollars, so US $35,000 a month. My family could afford it for nine months before they had to sell the house." Within a few hours of taking Trikafta, Jess had new energy, and within two weeks, her lung function increased 24%.

---

77. Svenja Espenhahn, "Advocating for Access to Orphan Drugs: Beth and Madison Vanstone's Story," *Canadian Rare Disease Network*, May 14, 2022. https://canadianrdn.ca/advocating-for-access-to-orphan-drugs-beth-and-madison-vanstones-story/
78. Jess's experience with having a family while on Trikafta was discussed in chapter 5.

While the changes in her health were remarkable, she knew that making her family homeless at the cost of her health was unjust. She decided to see if she could gain the support of citizens in her country to petition the Pharmaceutical Benefits Scheme (PBS) to cover the cost through the government. She began by posting on social media, which led to the creation of a petition to parliament. "The goal was 25,000 signatures in thirty days. I think we ended up with 55,000," she explained. Appearances on the news and in newspapers soon followed.[79] Within three months of her advocacy, she received a call from the minister of health who informed her that Trikafta was going to be added to the PBS. Jess concluded, "We took on the government, and we won. We have Trikafta. It was insane." Just like Beth and Madi in Canada, Jess's fortitude has led to countless people who they will never meet being able to live healthier lives. They are heroes—reminders that one person can make a difference.

Andrii Lukianets, who is forty years old, gained access to Trikafta another way. He grew up in Ukraine and had a milder form of CF compared to his sister, who died when she was twelve years old. During his teenage years, his health began to decline. "The disease gradually made itself . . . known more often," described Andrii. He had more frequent bouts of bronchitis, shortness of breath, and a cough that never went away. Multiple hospitalizations a year became a constant reality. In 2013, his lung collapsed, followed by a second and third experience of lung collapses. "The surgeons barely saved me," Andrii reflected. He had access to some medications in Ukraine to try to improve his health. Andrii explained, "We received Creon and Pulmozyme from the state budget, sometimes with interruptions, but we could only dream of targeted therapy [gene modulators]." In larger cities, like Kyiv and Lviv, access to antibiotics

---

79. Tita Smith, "Why this brave Aussie woman is forced to fork out $21,375 a MONTH just to survive after doctors warned she had six months to live—but she's running out of money fast," in *Daily Mail Australia*. February 22, 2022. https://www.dailymail.co.uk/news/article-10538711/Aussie-woman-living-cystic-fibrosis-forced-fork-21-375-MONTH-just-survive.html.

and inhalers was sometimes easier than where Andrii lived, but they also did not have access to gene modulators.

In his late thirties, Andrii's health grew worse: "I could not cope with the constant exacerbations in my lungs, and my general condition was worsening." As his health was failing, the continued costs of medications made life even more difficult. His lung function was at 16 and he was on oxygen throughout the day: "I had trouble even moving around my apartment . . . [and] I had to pay the costs of all the necessary intravenous antibiotic therapy due to a lack of funding in my city," Andrii explained. In the fall of 2021, he created a fundraiser to try to afford Trikafta on the "black market." He raised enough money to buy two months' worth of the medication and began taking it on February 20, 2022.

February 2022 is also significant because that is when Russia invaded Ukraine. "And then the war began, and I was forced to look for a way to survive," described Andrii. He was able to move to Austria "under the status of temporary protection," where he now has access to healthcare, including Trikafta. Since taking Trikafta, his lung function is up to 34% and he has not needed daily oxygen. His weight also increased from 62 kilograms to 89 kilograms. "I can walk and work without problems," he happily explained. "These results are amazing!" Andrii reflected about his Trikafta transformation: "I couldn't even imagine how much my condition would improve. If all patients had such access from childhood, I am sure they could live a full life." While the war has destroyed much of the life that Andrii knew, it has helped him gain access to a medication that has saved his life. His determination to seek protective status and to leave his home has given Andrii a future he never thought possible.

While completing this book, Suzy informed me that Andrea and her family had moved from Honduras to Spain so she would have access to Trikafta. "She is doing much better," Suzy expressed. I am grateful that her family was able to move, and I know that many people are unable to take this drastic action. Just as Jess's family was willing to sell their house, love may mean doing everything possible to help a child survive. Whether that means lobbying a government or moving across the world, sometimes advocacy for those in need is an extraordinary success.

The Next Frontier

I have traveled to Ecuador several times to work with a program called *Rostro de Cristo*, which primarily sends recent college graduates to live and work in marginalized communities abroad. During one of my trips, a volunteer told me something that one of her neighbors shared with a group of college students who had come to visit the country. She asked them to consider that human beings everywhere are much more similar than different. She then powerfully exclaimed, "The only difference between you and me is you were born under a different star." This image has stayed with me, not only because of its simple truth but also its cosmic vision. Every person could have been born in a different place, leading to a different set of opportunities, advantages, and disadvantages. I could have been born in Honduras, like the young man in the opening diary entry. Or, I could have been born in Ecuador, like this woman. In many other places in the world, CF would have been a death sentence when I was born. It has been for countless children who did not get access to the same medications and procedures I had when I was born, children who might still be alive today had they been born in a different country.

My friend Adem Riahi is twenty-four years old and lives in Tunisia. He knew little about what it meant to have cystic fibrosis growing up. Adem explained, "I didn't even take enzymes regularly because I didn't know what they did or why I was taking them." When he was fifteen, he learned more about the disease from doctors, as well as by looking up things on the Internet. He discovered that living with CF is a lifelong fight. As a teenager, he feared that his CF diagnosis would keep him from being able to complete his studies. Taking care of himself has helped him to stay healthy enough to maintain good grades and to keep learning. "I have achieved my dream because I am studying computer diagnostics of cars," he explained.

Adem knows that living each day with CF may be a struggle. "I live with the disease as if I were in a battle and one of us must win," he described. CF doesn't currently keep him from doing many things, but it does prevent him from boxing and Taekwondo, two activities he wishes he could do. Adem does a lot of things like other people his age, such as visiting his family and friends, going to coffee shops, and watching sports. He is also studying English. Adem's experience with CF is different from many of the people in this book. "There are not many treatments for maintaining health," he reflected. He is able to have IV medications when he gets really sick, but enzymes can be difficult to procure. He has a therapy vest thanks to *CF Vests Worldwide*, for which he is very grateful.

When it comes to gene modulators, Adem explained, "Doctors do not know much about Trikafta or Orkambi here." He is told by doctors that the low number of people with CF in Tunisia as well as the high cost [of the medication] would make getting access to Trikafta difficult, if not impossible. Adem implored, "I ask all patients to unite in one voice and help patients like us who are in poor countries to receive lifesaving medicines because we are truly dying here in silence. No one can hear us." There is no question that Adem deserves Trikafta just as much as I do. The country he lives in and the number of people in his country with CF does not diminish his human need for access to life-sustaining medication. The difference between me and my friend Adem isn't that one of us is more deserving to live. The difference is that he was born under a different star.

Roughly 7,000 kilometers east of Tunisia, a seven-year-old boy named Vihaan Krishna is growing up with CF in India. Vihaan's mother, Shwetha, loves her son dearly: "As his parent, watching him navigate this condition has been both heart-wrenching and inspiring." Vihaan enjoys acting and recreating movie scenes, as well as building with Legos and solving jigsaw puzzles. In 2023, Vihaan met some members of a movie team who were filming about a child with CF. His mother recalled, "The entire team met us, and they were both shocked and happy to meet a real-life CF warrior. . . . They were all excited and encouraged him to become a wonderful actor in the future."

Vihaan benefits from having doctors who know about CF as well as having access to some CF medications. However, his family must pay for all of them out-of-pocket: "Unfortunately, we don't have access to Trikafta in India. While we are happy to see other countries benefiting from it, we wish it were available here as well. Even if we tried to get it, the cost would be so high that most families wouldn't be able to afford it, even for a single month," explained Shwetha. Getting Trikafta could make a huge difference in Vihaan's future. Shwetha reflected, "Over the past four years I have seen far too many children with CF pass even before reaching their teenage years. If Trikafta were available here, it could give these children a real chance at a longer, better life, which they all deserve." Shwetha knows that Trikafta isn't the same as other medications: "Trikafta could drastically improve quality of life by addressing the underlying cause of CF," she explained. Her desire for her son to have the same chances for a happy and healthy life is evident in the way she speaks about him. Vihaan may one day follow his dreams and become a movie star or editor. His chances would be even greater if he had access to gene modulators.

During chaplain residency training, we gained awareness of our privilege and how it can be appropriately used in our care of others. I was unsure how this would appear until I found myself in the emergency room responding to a trauma during an evening shift. The hospital was on lockdown, which occurs when there has been a serious event where large crowds gather outside; the hospital limits who can come in, for the protection of patients. In this case, the patient was a child, and her mother was permitted to be with her daughter. The patient's mother became upset that her mother, the patient's grandmother, was not allowed to join her. "I need my mother here too," she said exasperatedly to the nurses and security. I told her I would speak to the doctor and advocate that an additional family member would be helpful. When I spoke with the doctor, she agreed and told me I could tell security that she supported the grandmother being present. The patient's mother was very grateful for my assistance. That evening, I came to see a dimension of the chaplain's role as a family advocate. It is a position of privilege that allowed me to move freely through the hospital, to speak on behalf of the patient's family. Access to Trikafta is similar. It is a position of privilege that allows me to move freely and is an invitation to speak on behalf of others who do not have the same luxury.

When I was young, I used to play with Legos and enjoyed doing puzzles, like Vihaan. I enjoy watching sports and hanging out with my friends, like Adem. If I were born in India or Tunisia, I would be like them, hoping that someday I could get access to the medication that I need to live longer. Perhaps acts of advocacy, like those of Beth, Madi, and Jess, in Canada and Australia, will someday make a difference for people in other countries. I know that people are dying in countries around the world where access to enzymes, inhalers, vests, and gene modulators is rare. I know that I have access to these treatments, and they help me to live longer. I also know that the only difference between me and them is that I was born under a different star.

Conclusion

Garden Justice

Injustice toward those with CF who are not experiencing the transformation of gene modulators comes in many forms. Some people are accused of lying or are verbally attacked for speaking the truth of their reality. Others feel excluded and forgotten, especially when their friends are the ones not recognizing their struggles. And sadly, there are also those who are not seen at all. My mentor, Fr. Howard Gray, SJ often told us, "The opposite of love isn't hate; it's indifference." Respecting human dignity means that no one is treated with indifference. Those who feel unheard need to be offered a microphone to speak; those who have been excluded need to be invited to the table, and those who are unseen need to be the guest of honor at the banquet of the gene modulator transformation. This is an image of celebrating garden justice.

Cheri Nel is no stranger to injustice. She is forty and lives in Johannesburg, South Africa. Cystic fibrosis primarily affected her pancreas until her twenties, when her lung function began to decline. She was aware, in 2010, of the upcoming development of gene modulators. Unfortunately, access to them in South Africa was elusive. When Trikafta was developed, she heard of the amazing transformations of those taking it. Cheri waited for Vertex and South Africa to come to an agreement for supplying it to the 500 people in her country who have CF. As time passed, many were forced to take an unapproved generic version developed in Argentina, called Trixacar. To get it, people flew from South Africa to Argentina to purchase it in person every six months.[80] It is less expensive, and

---

80. Kat Lay, "South Africans take on big pharma for access to 'miracle' cystic fibrosis drug," in *The Guardian*, March 18, 2024. https://www.theguardian.

some believe it is nearly as effective as Trikafta. Before taking it, Cheri took her PFT at 85%. Forty-eight hours after her first dose, her PFT increased to 105%.

Although she was feeling better on Trixacar, the difficulty acquiring it and the fact that many people in South Africa were not able to get it caused Cheri to take matters into her own hands. In early 2024, she sued Vertex to gain access to Trikafta, applying the Constitution of South Africa as her basis. The lawsuit accused Vertex of failing to make patented medication available on reasonable terms.[81] "My allegation was that Vertex is guilty of patient abuse and violating human rights," Cheri explained. She was surprised about how the media spread the word about what she was doing. "The combination of a lawsuit and the power of the media—that put a lot of pressure on Vertex," Cheri reflected. Before the trial against them started, Vertex created a program in South Africa that makes Trikafta accessible through a nonprofit organization that is supplying the money, which is coming from pharmaceutical companies around the world. "We didn't get to set a legal precedent, but we did get to set a commercial precedent," explained Cheri. "In South Africa you can slot in a different disease and different medication [into the court papers] and you don't have to do the background research, combine it with media, and maybe you will get a phenomenal result." The ingenuity and adaptation will look different in other countries, but Cheri's accomplishment stands as an example. "Maybe it will help someone, some way," she reflected.

Cheri has been on Trikafta since August 2023 and is excited to be able to spend many more years with her partner and work as an investment banker. Living with a chronic disease has taught her that tomorrow isn't promised: "I am all about the here and the now," she explained. "Take the maximum out of life. . . . The bad cards that were dealt to you . . . could be your key advantage in

---

com/global-development/2024/mar/18/cystic-fibrosis-patient-south-africa-cheri-nel-lawsuit-big-pharma-generic-drugs-trikafta-access-vertex.

81. Kat Lay, "South Africans take on big pharma for access to 'miracle' cystic fibrosis drug."

life. Getting a bad hand doesn't mean you are out of the game. Play as best you can." Cheri's ingenuity and advocacy are examples of not only playing the hand that she is dealt but passing a card to those around her, lifting them up, so they have a chance to play the game. Her efforts have given a microphone to those unheard, a seat at the table to those who were told there is no place for them, and now 500 people in South Africa are going to attend the gene modulator banquet as guests of honor. Cheri has tilled the soil of garden justice so seeds of today can become roses tomorrow.

Part Four

Fragrance of a Rose

I was introduced to the study of theology around the time that I was "introduced" to my chronic illness. I was not raised in an overly religious household but became curious about different concepts of God, faith, and religion. Following high school, I double-majored in history and religious studies at John Carroll University and remained there to complete an MA in religious studies. Two years later, I accepted an assistantship at Duquesne University, where I completed my PhD in systematic theology. The more I learned, the less I felt I knew. Chaplaincy served as a capstone to my previous theological studies. The content I learned in class came alive nearly every visit, regardless of the patient's religiosity. The dynamic between hope and suffering was often prevalent as the patients taught me to sit with the tension between those two concepts.

Part Four will explore theological paradigms, perspectives on hope, and the wisdom that grows from the fertile soil of chronic illness. Throughout the book, the roses have been speaking. They have told their stories, reflecting on their growth and hardships. In Part Four, the words of the roses turn into an invitation to question how their experiences touch one's heart. The fragrance of the roses is a gift to the world. I hope paying attention to these words can be a bouquet that delights your soul and invites you to "spin with joy."

Chapter 10

Where Is the Divine?

I keep praying for a cure. I feel like God isn't an-
swering me and I don't understand why. I try to be
a good person and to be nice to others. I don't know
why I have this genetic disease while all my friends
are healthy. Am I being punished for something my
parents did? If so, is that fair? I'll keep praying, but
I am losing hope and faith that God will help me.
Maybe there isn't a God at all. Goodnight.

Despite the overwhelming presence of suffering in the world, many people believe in a higher power or supreme being. Most of those people believe that this *being*, often referred to as God, has some control over causing, or at least, ceasing, this suffering. There have been many books written, from various religious perspectives, on the issue of theodicy, or why evil and suffering exist concurrently with a supposedly all-powerful and all-good deity. This chapter will not primarily focus on philosophical arguments. Instead, it will expound on the interplay between hope and suffering by sharing reflections on how faith may play a role in the life of a person with a chronic illness, as well as through some of my experiences as a hospital chaplain sitting with people wrestling with religious questions. I did not ask a question on religion in the interviews. If people brought up their faith, I invited them to explore their perspectives more deeply. One should not take this to mean that everyone I spoke to was religious. Each person mentioned in this book has a unique perspective on faith and/or God in the face of suffering and mortality. I think this diversity is a strength, not a weakness, and is something to be celebrated.

Holy Ground

Midway through my residency, a middle-aged male patient requested to see a chaplain because he was trying to find a former pastor. I went into the visit expecting to be given a name to search for online. What I found was a veteran whose chart indicated his body was decimated with cancer, including brain cancer that left him barely intelligible. He repeated the pastor's name multiple times until I had it correct. I informed him that I would try my best to find him, sensing this man did not have much time left to live. He then requested I pray with him. He extended his shaking and brittle hands, and I held them in my own. I closed my eyes and began to pray. When I opened them, I saw tears flowing down his cheeks and noticed that my eyes had also become wet. The man tried to say "thank you" as he stuttered to get the words out. He then drew my hands to his mouth and kissed them. I was so touched by his action that I clutched his hands even tighter. A few moments later he released my hands, and I began to slowly back out of the room. His last words to me were, "Pray for me that he [God] takes me quickly."

When I left the room, despite feeling sad and powerless, I also felt lighter, as though I was glowing. I think I felt this way because in that moment I was touched by the divine grace of this dying man. The innocence of his kiss on my hands, the tears we shared, and his total reliance on the Divine, knowing that he had reached the end of his life, made this a powerful moment. There were a few visits that I had during my time as a chaplain where I felt this presence of the Spirit, often when I was with people who I felt were prophets or messengers of God—people who have come to understand their time is short and that their encounter with the Divine or eternity is near. This is a fate that we all will face. The question is how prepared will we be when our time comes?

In the Introduction, I cited Brené Brown's observation that "stories are data with a soul." I believe the sharing of this data, these stories, is always a spiritual experience. By spiritual I mean that stories invite us to sit with realities of the human condition that are beyond space and time, touching common human experiences.

This does not mean that every story is religious. People telling their stories can choose to interpret or experience their lives through a religious or theological lens. Reading this book, like reading other books with stories, invites you to examine your own story, emotions, or feelings. Perhaps a person you met within these pages caused you to think of a loved one who lives with a chronic illness, or who has died. Perhaps you saw something in another's reflections that touched some of your own story. This experience of going beyond the present moment into your memory or imagination is what I am calling a spiritual experience.

For some people, the spiritual experience is also a religious one. The man who was dying of brain cancer requested that I offer a prayer at his bedside. He appeared to believe in a God who could hear this prayer or be present in a powerful way. I would like to suggest that the moment I shared with him in the room became *holy ground*. I do not mean that it had been officially blessed by an ordained religious person, which is how something becomes "holy" in many religious traditions. Rather, I mean it became a place where humans shared a spiritual or divine experience of God's presence.

Sonja Petrovic had an experience of holy ground. In 2018, she was preparing for surgery to remove part of her lung. She was sitting in her room listening to worship music, scared about the uncertainty of what would come. Suddenly, she felt a sense of peace. She used her phone to take a selfie to capture the moment. The peace she felt internally is evident from the picture. "It [the picture] reminds me that there is that peace that surpasses all understanding," she reflected. "In that moment, I surrendered everything and I was like, 'Okay God . . . whatever happens, you are in control.'" Like my experience with the man dying from cancer, this feeling seemed to come from beyond her—a sense of peace, given to her on holy ground.

She was extubated following the procedure, but her heart stopped, and she was re-intubated. During the following year, she fought for her life as her lung function dropped to 26%. Without the surgery, she would have died right away. With the surgery, she still had to struggle to survive . . . until she began taking

Trikafta. Sonja reflected on this transition: "I was getting ready to go on oxygen and I was blessed with Trikafta, which completely changed the game for me, changed my life." She felt the physical results the next day, while pulling herself from the "disability mindset" took much longer. She had been so prepared to die that she "was afraid to live, not knowing what is expected." Her faith has played a huge role in navigating this transition.

Sonja views her new life as a gift from God. She prayed to live long enough to see her children grow up, and now she has been blessed with three grandchildren. She affirmed with honesty, "Whatever happens from here, I have lived the fullest life, beyond not just my life expectancy, but beyond my own expectations." In response to this gift, Sonja tries to live the most loving life possible: "I know that is why I'm put on this Earth, to show the love of Christ, and just to be a light to others, . . . to be a beacon of light, because I know there are so many people who are hurting." Transforming her struggle into love for others is a powerful mission, one supported by the peaceful embrace of the Spirit of God, found in the holy ground of her hospital room.

"It was the first time I realized that the peace of God is a real thing," recalled Maude Perrine, a Jehovah's Witness. Maude felt God's presence when she was five or six years old, following a ski accident. Her father offered to pray with her prior to the operation. Like Sonja, Maude recalls feeling a sense of peace unlike any she had felt before: "Ever since then I just couldn't deny that he [God] was there with me, with every hospital stay." Maude, who grew up in Gatineau, Quebec, and now lives in Antigonish, Nova Scotia with her husband, is no stranger to hospitals. She was diagnosed with CF at the age of four, diabetes at eleven, and cepacia at thirteen. Maude reflected, "I was pretty much just waiting to die."

In her early twenties, her life changed when she began taking Trikafta. She offered, "Applying for jobs was super weird. . . . I'm in my twenties and it's the first time in my life that I am looking for work—never thought that would be a thing." She has more energy and is now planning trips with her husband unencumbered by her medical equipment. It has been strange for Maude to compare her previous life to this one: "You look back, so many things that you used to have to do or that you got used to being part of your life. And then you take Trikafta and it's not your life anymore. How easily you forget all those things."

Following Trikafta, Maude feels that despite all she has gained, she has lost one thing. That dependence on God's presence, from the time praying with her father when she was a child, is no longer as prominent. "So that is something I find I kind of miss. . . . I have to pay attention to the way God is in my life versus just having the whole other [experience] intensely," she confessed. When one has a powerful religious experience around illness, it can be hard to have the same religious fervor when the illness subsides. Maude doesn't regret taking Trikafta. She is looking for a way to have the same connection with God now that her life has been transformed. Maude is looking for a way to find holy ground in the everydayness that accompanies transformation, from waiting to die to actively living.

In their book, *The Spirituality of Imperfection*, Ernest Kurtz and Katherine Ketcham offer a helpful story to further explore the concept of holy ground:

> Time before time, when the world was young, two brothers shared a field and a mill. Each night they divided evenly the grain they had ground together during the day. Now, as it happened, one of the brothers lived alone; the other had a wife and a large family. One day, the single brother thought to himself: "It isn't really fair that we divide the grain evenly. I have only myself to care for, but my brother has children to feed." So each night he secretly took some of his grain to his brother's granary to see that he was never without.

> But the married brother said to himself one day, "It isn't really fair that we divide the grain evenly, because I have children to provide for me in my old age, but my brother has no one. What will he

do when he is old?" So every night he secretly took some of his grain to his brother's granary. As a result, both of them always found their supply of grain mysteriously replenished each morning.

Then one night the brothers met each other halfway between their two houses, suddenly realized what had been happening, embraced each other in love. The story is that God witnessed their meeting and proclaimed, "This is a holy place—a place of love—and here it is that my temple shall be built." And so it was. The holy place, where God is made known, is the place where human beings discover each other in love.[82]

The Spirituality of Imperfection uses stories to help make meaning out of life, especially in cases where people are ensnared by the belief that without perfection, their lives are diminished. I have always enjoyed this story about holy ground because it demonstrates that a place can be made holy through encounter. I am not discounting the importance of blessing in religious traditions; I am offering a way to reframe holiness. For Sonja and Maude, where they encountered peace became holy ground.

Mark Bettinger understands his CF journey and the suffering he has gone through using the lens of eternity. "My lung disease has taken me to a deeper intimacy with Christ that I don't think anything else could have," he reflected, in a similar way to Maude. Two years before Mark's birth, his brother died from CF, so his parents were aware of how terminal CF can be. Mark's health, however, was pretty stable until he was seventeen years old. He began having yearly IV antibiotics for the next few years. In 2004, he got married and he and his wife had children using IVF. Around 2014 or 2015, his health began to decline rapidly. His lung function declined to 26% and he was referred to the lung transplant team in

82. Ernest Kurtz and Katherine Ketcham, *The Spirituality of Imperfection: Storytelling and the Search for Meaning* (Bantam Books, 1993), 9–10.

St. Louis. Apparently, Orkambi was causing his lung function to decline, and once doctors took him off it, his lung function went back up to 40%. Symdeko did not have a positive effect either; it appeared that nothing would stave off his decline.

In November 2019, Mark began taking Trikafta. It has helped a number of his CF side effects but has also resulted in a catch-22. While his lung function increased to 51% following Trikafta, he developed constant pain: "My lung capacity increased, but in terms of quality of life, [and] pain, that has deteriorated pretty substantially." He and his doctors discussed the balance of Trikafta stabilizing his lung function and giving him energy with the tradeoff of the pain from the lung inflammation that they say isn't normal. Mark concluded, "I am willing to live with the pain increase. . . . I'm willing to pay." Mark wants to live to see his kids grow up.

Mark credits his faith with helping him deal with his illness and constant pain. "I came to Christ when I was six [years old] after my mom was killed in a car accident with my brother. I was with my dad in the vehicle in front of them on an interstate headed to Iowa," he recalled. That left him living with his father, a single parent of a child who was told he would not live beyond eighteen. A year later, he began going to church with the woman who became his stepmom. That is where he "came to Christ." Mark explained, "I came to Christ when I heard the message that Jesus loves you and that he died for you." During his adult life, Mark has been able to follow that call as a missionary because of Trikafta: "It is . . . because of two yellow pills and a blue pill I take with 10 grams of fat every day." Mark described how CF has demonstrated to him the importance of surrendering to Christ every day: "CF has taught me to depend on God and not . . . on myself, to trust him with my life." He is grateful that he can continue to follow God's will with whatever time he has left. Mark uses his experience and loss to create holy ground through his work as a missionary and with a loving family—the holy place where God is made known, the place where human beings encounter each other in love.

Encountering another person in love has special meaning for those who have had a lung transplant. Dylan Mortimer grew up surrounded by religion, as his father was a pastor.[83] From this foundation, he has continued to explore his religious beliefs through his art, friendships, and transplants. Dylan described a theological connection to receiving an organ as the ultimate gift: "It is very much like the Gospel to me. I . . . needed someone to give me lungs that I couldn't give to myself. . . . And . . . you cannot repay that. I can't go give somebody else my lungs. It is really very humbling. I didn't earn or deserve that." The gift of life that he carries around in his body reminds him that his life has been given to him. The story of the two brothers sharing grain takes on a different significance when the "grain" is an organ that they both need to survive. The description of holy ground, however, remains the same. God is made known as Dylan received life, taking the ultimate gift from someone who chose to be an organ donor. As the Christian Gospel proclaims, life coming from death allows Dylan to live longer and to continue to share his CF story through his art.

Can God?

During my chaplain residency, I met with the mother of a patient who was dying of breast cancer. The patient was in her forties, and her mother requested to see a chaplain. I went into the visit with trepidation, expecting her to be angry at the injustice of watching her daughter die from cancer. I soon realized it was more confusion than anger that she was carrying. She tearfully described how people in her religious community had offered pedantic responses of trusting in God and God's plan to assuage her pain. She was looking for another way to understand how a loving God could exist, as she watched her daughter suffer. She had a powerful religious experience earlier in her life, and professed that she did not currently doubt that a God existed; however, she feared that when her daughter died, that previous divine moment may not be enough

---

83. Dylan's ability to share his CF story through art was previously described in the Introduction.

to offset the agony and anger of her loss. Ultimately, her question wasn't "*Does* God exist?" It was "What *sort* of God exists?"

Those in Western religious traditions (Jews, Christians, and Muslims) wrestle with the tension between a seemingly powerful God and the prevalence of evil and suffering in the world. These are important questions for believers as well as philosophers. As my residency educator, Ron Cooper, pointed out, "When prayer doesn't go our way, we never see God the same." The work of exploring the question of God's attributes, and how those images affect our lives, can rise to the surface of our consciousness, especially during times of illness and duress. These images of God play a central role in one's relationship with God. This may be especially true for those who live with a chronic illness.

Kari Rose shared how having CF affected her relationship with God growing up.[84] "At first, I was really mad at God," Kari reflected on her teenage years. "I didn't understand how people are saying we serve this loving, gracious God, and here I am, with this completely broken body from birth—from conception." Kari explains that she really struggled with her identity as a Christian. As she has gotten older, she has focused more on the blessings in her life: "There is no way I would be here if it wasn't for God." She described the way scientists and researchers continue to come up with treatments for illnesses, and that those people are using the intelligence God gave them. "That all comes from God. God created those people to be able to do those things and to have the desire to do those things," she explained. She still struggles from time to time with being angry, though: "Sometimes my head doesn't always agree with what my heart feels."

Kari's processing of anger mirrors the feelings and doubts of the mother whose daughter was dying from cancer. Like Kari, she was angry and looking for a way to understand. Why would a loving God give Kari a "body broken from birth" any more than God would cause this woman's daughter to have a body riddled with cancer in the prime years of her life? I felt similar sentiments in the months

---

84. Kari's experience with post-Trikafta reality was described in chapter 6.

following my reading of the *Blueprint* article on Mr. Luedeke. The diary entry that introduced this chapter would have been written toward the end of my first year in high school. I had recently learned that having CF would likely preclude me from joining the Jesuits, a Catholic religious order known for working with the marginalized. My religious development was in its nascent stage, and I had become enthralled with the vision of living in an impoverished community and working for justice. I felt that God was calling me to dedicate my life to these endeavors. Learning that CF was a terminal illness, and that it could keep me from being a Jesuit, was a double blow in the early stages of my religious development.

For a year, I wanted nothing to do with religion. The anger I felt that God had created me as "broken," seemed unfair. From conception, I had an incurable disease that would prevent me from living a life of helping others. I felt shame for not being able to do things, and thought it was unjust for God to have done this "to me." I often prayed, "God, I don't want a cure for me. I want a cure so I can help others." Eventually, I came to terms with my limitations and grew in my understanding of my relationship with God. As I tell my students, I didn't go into studying theology because I knew what I believed about God. I went into studying theology because I wanted to learn *what* I believed about God. Being exposed to numerous philosophies and theologies has been formative and helpful as I applied this understanding in the real-world setting of hospital chaplaincy. That does not mean I have figured out the answer to theodicy. It means I have figured out *my* answer, one that allows me to affirm belief in God while acknowledging suffering. It is an answer that helps me give meaning to life and is always open to new lessons taught to me by students, patients, the world, and the Divine.

Another person who echoed similar sentiments of religious anger is Alexa Ciancimino.[85] Like Kari, she was angry at God during her teenage years. She explained, "I was really in a dark place. I was depressed all the time. I was angry. . . . My relationship with God

---

85. Alexa's positive experience with Trikafta was described in chapter 5 through her analogy of winning the lottery.

was horrible. I was just like, God hates me." It is understandable how a young person who is saddled with daily medical treatments that her friends do not have to do can conclude that God doesn't love her. When Alexa had her first discussion about lung transplants with doctors, she had a panic attack. While discussing transplants, one medical person told her, "Just keep in mind that you won't live very long after the transplant." Alexa recalls staying up the whole night crying: "It just became harder to really see into the future. . . . I couldn't plan anything." Alexa saw her possibility for a future vanishing, as her faith in God was doing the same.

Alexa's relationship with God took another difficult turn when her boyfriend Jeffrey died, in August 2022. Jeffrey also had CF, a rarity for two people with CF to attempt a relationship. Jeffrey had a lung transplant, but he started getting chronic rejection. His death made Alexa's relationship with God rockier. She explained, "It is like any relationship. There are ups and downs. Even with God, sometimes we are not on speaking terms." Despite this dynamic, Alexa still prays every day and is grateful for the blessing that Trikafta has been for her life. She has also created a nonprofit organization to help honor Jeffrey. *Jeffrey's House* is dedicated to giving financial support to families whose loved one is having a transplant in the Bay Area. It is her way of trying to create life from death.

Alexa's grandfather recently sent her, *When Bad Things Happen to Good People*, by Rabbi Harold Kushner. She explained, "I thought when I was younger God gave me this disease for some reason. He [God] just wants me to be miserable. But then I read that book, [and] he [Kushner] said God doesn't do this to us. It is just a fact of life." Kushner expresses that it is up to human beings to decide how to approach suffering and tragedy. Alexa continued, "What God does is allow us to give meaning to even the worst situation." Alexa's nonprofit is a great example of how inspiration can come from death and loss.

Ironically, that book played an important role in my theological exploration when I read it in college. At the time, I felt that God decided to give me CF, a view that I no longer hold. Kushner writes,

"God does not cause our misfortunes. Some are caused by bad luck, some are caused by bad people, and some are simply an inevitable consequence of our being human and being mortal, living in a world of inflexible natural laws."[86] Kushner continues that God is not punishing people, nor is our suffering part of God's grand plan. God does play an important role in the world for Kushner. He writes, "God, who neither causes nor prevents tragedies, helps by inspiring people to help."[87] If Kushner is correct, it would mean not only did God not pick me to have CF, but it would also mean God could not have prevented me from having CF.

A book from Christian author, Thomas Oord, offers a similar response to the problem of evil. In his book, *God Can't*, Oord offers a model of God that falls outside traditional Christian theologies, as Kushner does with his interpretation of Judaism. Oord writes, "It doesn't make sense to say a loving God *permits* evil. We don't need to say, 'Your rape happened for a reason,' and mean 'God allowed it.' We don't need to believe God allows children to be tortured or think God permits cancer. And so on. We can believe painful experiences and horrific tragedies make the world worse than it might have been. And God didn't want them. Ultimately, evil is evil . . . from God's perspective and ours."[88] Oord concludes that God *can't* prevent these things from happening. God doesn't decide to allow evil that could be prevented because that would go against God's nature of love. Oord explains, "When I say God 'can't' prevent evil, I mean God is unable to control people, other creatures, or circumstances that cause evil."[89] Oord refers to this concept as God's "uncontrolling love" that is part of God's nature.

Although Oord and Kushner explain their ideas differently, I believe they are approaching the problem of evil in the same way.

---

86. Harold S. Kushner, *When Bad Things Happen to Good People* (Avon Books, 1981), 134.
87. Kushner, 140.
88. Thomas Jay Oord, *God Can't: How to Believe in God and Love after Tragedy, Abuse and Other Evils* (Sacra-Sage Press, 2019), 13.
89. Oord, *God Can't*, 27.

They are placing limits on what God can do in ways that traditional Jewish, Christian, and Muslim theologies refuse to do. While it may help explain evil as something that is uncaused, it shifts the theological focus to exploring a new definition of God's power, a movement most believers in Western theistic traditions prefer not to do. Whether you agree or disagree with this approach, I think it is important to decide what role God has in evil. Does God cause specific people to have horrible diseases? If so, why? Is it punishment for something they did or did not do? If God does not cause illness but could prevent it, is that morally better or worse than believing God caused it? And finally, how does your answer affect your image of, or relationship with, God?

One place where Kushner, Oord, and many traditional believers agree is that the world is a place of suffering. Rachel Meddaugh sees CF as confirmation of the suffering and brokenness of the world. At four years old, Rachel received a feeding tube, which she had for the next eleven years. In her teenage years, she heard about a fourteen-year-old girl who died from CF. Rachel recalls, "But for me it was like, oh wait, she has what I have. And she is younger than me . . . and that was hard to grapple with." Rachel came to terms with CF Time in a powerful way.

In 2020, Rachel began taking Trikafta, following her senior year in high school. She recalls, "And I remember the first day I took the pills, my heart was pounding, and I was home from college. I went to the beach and just sat there." She began coughing up a lot of mucus, undergoing the purge. Rachel thoughtfully reflected, "My body was cleansing itself and finally working partly the way it was designed to work." In the weeks ahead, her cough decreased, and she had more energy.

Rachel believes that the experience of those with CF and other chronic illnesses is a theological sign that the world is not perfect. She reflected, "CF affirms creation's longing for redemption and healing. . . . I am living testimony that the world is broken, and things aren't perfect right now." Some forms of Christian theology would identify this as "garden theology", calling to mind the reality that life on this side of the garden of Eden is imperfect. Whether one believes that the garden of Eden story in Genesis is historical or mythical, one theological lesson from the story is that the world is not as God intended. Rachel's body works a bit more like it was intended, but it will never work fully on this side of the garden. It is the hope of many religions that there is a state of existence where it will.

Like Western religions, Eastern religions and philosophies also offer perspectives on suffering and evil. Buddhism speaks of suffering and its predominant role in life. One of the core teachings in Buddhist philosophy are the four noble truths. These are: life is suffering, the cause of suffering, the cessation of suffering, and the 8-fold path.[90] Buddhism affirms that suffering comes from trying to hold on to what is not permanent. For example, clinging to money, power, physical beauty, or the many other things that can be fleeting. When we lose those things, we suffer, because we believe they can be retained. The well-known author Thich Nhat Hanh's first chapter of his book, *Being Peace,* is entitled "Suffering is not Enough."[91] Hanh attempts to reframe the four noble truths by offering that we can see the world as suffering, or, we can decide that there is more to life than suffering. Hanh affirms that love and understanding can be greater than the suffering we experience. Recalling Kushner and Oord, love becomes the predominant antidote to living in a broken world. I encourage people of any religious background to read some of Hanh's work, not to replace their religious views, but to supplement them with a philosophy based on treating others with love and respect. These reflections may offer new perspectives on where the Divine is, especially when living with a chronic disease.

The most difficult night of my residency began with a conversation with an elderly man in the ICU. He indicated he was getting stronger and hoped to be moved to a step-down unit. He identified as Catholic, although mentioned his religious views were varied.

---

90. Houston Smith, *The World's Religions* (HarperCollins Publishers, 1991), 99–103.
91. Thich Nhat Hanh, *Being Peace* (Parallax Press, 1987), 13–16.

As I left his room he asked me, "Chaplain, why does God take children?" We both paused under the weight of his theological inquiry. He then broke the silence, "I don't want you to answer it. Just think about it." The teacher in me wanted to delve into the question, and invite him to unpack what he meant by "take" and to look at different perspectives of God's relationship to the world. The chaplain in me realized the old man was growing tired and was having coughing fits between his sentences. I decided to leave the question for another time and wished him a goodnight.

Up until that evening, I had not had an experience as a chaplain ministering to a dying child. Two hours after this man's penetrating question, I was called to the emergency room. Two children had been hit by a car when they ran into the street without looking. One survived and would recover. The other child was in critical condition in a coma. This child died a few days later. This was the most heartbreaking experience of my chaplain residency. I will never forget the wailing of tears when the family heard the next day that their little girl was brain-dead.

The child's parents tried to convince themselves that all would be okay. It was their way of grieving the horror they were facing. I did the best I could to be present to them while the voice of the man in the ICU danced in my mind like raindrops striking a metal surface, scattering in all directions. I felt unequipped and unprepared. No religion or philosophy, no ancient texts or bestsellers, prepare you for that moment. It was as though this man was a prophet foreshadowing what was to come. Chaplain, why does God take children?

I do not have an answer for why God "takes" children any more than I have an answer for why I have CF. It can be consoling to think that God gave me this disease for a greater purpose or that God saved the first child. It helped to soften the anger of my youth. However, knowing that would mean that one child was ordained to die makes this perspective less acceptable. These realities make me conclude that the answer I held in my youth is incongruent with my current image of God. It is not my place to decide what God can, or cannot, do, nor is it my agenda to convince readers of this book how to approach theodicy. I simply offer, for those who believe in a higher power, that it is important to reflect on what your personal theology says about God's role in tragedy. Asking these questions from a place of freedom and security, rather than desperation and need, may help that reconciliation when the time comes. As my residency educator, Ron Cooper, told us many times, "We are all just one accident or illness away from being that person in the hospital bed." Such is life on this side of the garden.

Chapter 11

The Thing with Feathers

Someday, people won't die from CF the way they do now. They won't have to live life grasping for moments in their teenage years, uncertain if they will reach midlife. CF will be something they forget unless it is brought up at a routine doctor's checkup. I may not live long enough to see this day, but those born today with CF will have a different life from mine. They will have more opportunities, less hindered by a deteriorating body. That is why we advocate. That is why we support CF research. That is why we hope. Goodnight.

Hope can be a powerful weapon against fear. It can sustain people during difficult times and prepare people for the end of their lives, as they hope for something beyond this world. For those with a chronic illness, hope and a positive mindset may give strength to live beyond a diagnosis timetable or acceptance that the end is near, knowing they will continue to exist in the hearts of others. This chapter will explore hope through the contours of Emily Dickinson's famous poem *"Hope" is the thing with feather*s. Hope is something that can touch all people. At the same time, I have observed many situations of suffering and death as a chaplain where optimistic messages may not be congruent with everyone's life experience. These stories of hope are about honoring the dead, being inspired by the living, and looking to a time in the future when CF parents are not routinely told at their child's birth that the disease is terminal. Such a time is something for which we can all hope.

Perching in the Soul

My memory of awakening to CF Time and my truncated life expectancy while reading about Mr. Luedeke is immortalized in my soul. Until CPE, I had not given this moment the weight that it deserves. My self-exploration during chaplaincy training helped me to bring the blurriness of these early CF moments to clarity. Our life experiences, moments of triumph and tragedy, are sometimes undervalued when they happen. They may remain in the background of our subconscious, affecting our decisions and interactions for the rest of our lives. That morning, in March 1996, is one of those moments for me, waiting, or perching, in my soul until the time I was able to accept the way it was woven into the fabric of my life. I never met Mr. Luedeke, nor have I met anyone in his family. I never read anything he wrote, nor saw a video of him speaking. However, while writing this book, I have come to see him as a major influence on my life. While learning about Mr. Luedeke revealed to me that my time was short, he also demonstrated to me that I could overcome CF and become a teacher. His gift to me, someone he never met, was to teach me to follow my dreams in the time I had left.

Brynn Baskin never met her uncle Bruce just as I never met Mr. Luedeke. I met Brynn, who does not have CF, on a retreat. I spoke about my CF experience and played the song "I Lived" by One Republic. She approached me with her eyes full of tears and told me that her uncle Bruce had died from CF. She also explained how "I Lived" makes her think of her uncle because the official music video is about CF. I was touched that my CF story had connected to her life. Brynn later informed me that Bruce was born in 1958, when doctors were just coming to understand the disease. CF did not keep Bruce from living the fullest life possible. He had a family, went to law school, and always wanted people to treat him like a person who was not burdened by his disease. Around the time gene modulators were in the experimental stage, Bruce underwent a lung transplant. He never left the hospital and died four months later.

Even though Brynn was born two months after her uncle died, she feels her life guided by his spirit partly because she was named

Brynn Lea in honor of him, Bruce Lee. Every year she volunteers at the family's Bruce Baskin Golf Outing in Cleveland, Ohio, named in honor of her uncle. Her family also organizes other fundraisers for CF research. These events have inspired Brynn to want a career helping others, which she hopes to do by majoring in early childhood education. Brynn also gains courage during difficult times when she thinks of her uncle. She explained, "I guess that is one of the biggest lessons that I have learned from my dad, who learned it from my uncle, 'Don't let what people say affect you. . . . Let it roll off your back like a duck.'" She recently got a tattoo that says "Be a duck" to remind her to let things go. Brynn smiled and explained that the sentiment means to "live your life the way you want to. Just go at it however you want to live. It means a lot to me." Her uncle Bruce could have lived life as a sick child and listened to what society told him he couldn't do. Instead, he chose to live life to the fullest. As the One Republic song states, Bruce wanted to be able to say at the end of his life, "I lived." Brynn plans to embody this message, as the call to be a duck is perched on her soul by a role model she never met.

While Brynn and I never met our CF role models, Victoria DiSorbo's CF inspiration was her best friend growing up. Victoria does not have CF, like her childhood friend, Julie. Julie and Victoria met at the community pool when Julie's father moved to the United States from Belgium. Julie was around twelve years old, three years older than Victoria. Although she did not speak English, and Victoria did not speak Flemish, they immediately hit it off. Overcoming the language barrier, they spent time together nearly every day. One day, Victoria's parents explained to her that Julie had cystic fibrosis. Victoria recalls her parents telling her, "She has to do treatments and take medication whenever she eats. She may have to take it easy sometimes and may be in the hospital. . . . If you are going to continue this friendship, that is fine. You just need to know you will need to be selfless." The decision to grow closer to Julie, rather than to run away, remains a life-altering choice in Victoria's life.

In 2015, Julie returned to Belgium as her lung function had dropped to 20%. In February 2016, she went into surgery for a double lung transplant. Although her lungs took, her heart was unable to handle the transplant. She died a short time after the surgery. Victoria emotionally recalled the last time she saw Julie before she left for Belgium. "I was so stressed out," she tearfully shared, "She kept making me laugh. She never wanted to talk about the negative. She wanted to keep laughing, keep dancing, keep talking about the positive." Victoria described Julie as "the strongest person I ever had the pleasure of knowing. . . . She always lit up the room."

Julie's friendship profoundly affected Victoria. She became aware of Julie's CF needs in her teenage years and was inspired by the way she carried her disease. The influence not only formed her way of seeing the world, it also informed her life path. Before Julie died, Victoria, who was the shyer and more reserved of the duo, entered a beauty pageant so she could win the crown for Julie. To her surprise, she won and gave her the crown in the hospital, one of the last times she got to see her. At the end of 2015, Victoria entered Miss Teen USA recognizing that pageants were a vehicle for advocacy for CF. She placed in the top sixteen. A few months after Julie's death, Victoria decided to apply for another pageant, again advocating for a greater awareness around CF and to honor Julie's memory. She won Miss Florida Teen USA in October 2016 and, eventually, Miss World America in 2023. In 2024, she was in the top twenty in the Miss World competition, where she was able to speak about CF and healthcare to over three million people.

Victoria's advocacy beyond the pageant world and work with the *CF Foundation* keeps Julie's memory alive. Victoria explained, "Whenever I want to quit, or whenever I question myself, or whenever I think something is too big to achieve, I think of Julie." While continuing to advocate on an international stage, Victoria also hopes to become a mentor for young women with a chronic disease. Her courage comes from having an "angel on her shoulder," her friend Julie, who is perched on her soul, giving her strength to do more than she thinks is possible.

Like Victoria, my friend Marcos Gonzales holds a special connection to someone who has died from CF. Marcos' nephew,

Xavier, battled CF for fourteen years before his death on April 9, 2016. Xavier was diagnosed with CF during his first year of life. When Xavier was five years old, Marcos was in Jesuit formation, a time of study that offered him freedom to see his nephew. Marcos reflected on a time his sister and Xavier came to see him in Chicago during these studies. He shared, "When they came to visit, I . . . had a fixed mindset. We had to get to the train. . . . I remember rushing us, maybe two blocks . . . what seems for me a very innocuous activity. Seeing him once we got to the train, because of how fast I made us walk, and him significantly out of breath, was . . . eye-opening to me." Moved by Xavier's shortness of breath and his realization of the gift of having strong and healthy lungs, Marcos took up running.

Marcos was also able to deepen his relationship with his nephew when Xavier was able to come out to some of his races. "I would write his name on my arm, . . . and he got to join me [in that way] and be part of my running journey," Marcos explained, holding back tears. When doctors decided he needed a lung transplant, Xavier told Marcos the first thing he wanted to do with his new lungs was to run a marathon. Sadly, he never got the chance. A few months following the transplant, Xavier's lungs experienced increased complications, eventually leading to his death.

Before his death, Xavier told his mother the message he wished the world to hear was "have faith and be positive." Like Julie's last words to Victoria, Xavier left the world with a message of hope. People who could have been angry at living a short life chose to love and find positivity in their final moments. This outlook has likewise given Marcos a perspective on life. He emotionally explained to me, "I think the gift is realizing I had a longing to be a dad through the way I was loving Xavier. It was a large part of what helped me see I was called to fatherhood, not the priesthood. And that journey is one I have been on ever since in terms of being able to have the courage to make a difficult life decision." Marcos discerned and left the Jesuits not long after Xavier's death. It is very possible that someday Marcos will have a child, a life that may not exist if not for the courageous life of Xavier—a powerful example of life arising from death.

Marcos continues to run in Xavier's memory. In his early days of running, he worked with the *CF Foundation* in Chicago and raised $25,000. Now, he hopes to do a 100 miler and to continue raising money for CF research. When Xavier was preparing for his lung transplant, Marcos knew the gene modulator research would be too late to benefit Xavier, but he continued to raise money. He explained, "It would benefit others, and that is what we want. We want a cure." Marcos tearfully offered, "If I could run a mile and give him another day of life, I would not stop running. . . . I run because he couldn't, and I run because now he can, with me." Like Brynn, Marcos has a tattoo dedicated to his loved one. It is the EKG of Xavier's heartbeat from when he was healthy, scrolling down his forearm. Whether it is the wisdom of a duck, or the pulse of the heart, Brynn, Victoria, and Marcos have found ways to carry their loss.

Neither Brynn, Victoria, nor Marcos have CF, but loved ones who have died from the disease are part of their story. I have often heard this from friends and patients who have lost people to horrible diseases. A way to honor a deceased loved one is to treasure their memory, share stories, and be inspired by the life they lived. Emily Dickinson's poem speaks of the birdsong continuing to sing from within. The soul is the home of hope, the place it perches, never leaving. The roses do not need to be alive to speak. One can often hear their song long after they have died.

Sore Must Be the Storm

Rylee Walker stared out into the darkness in June 2023 with a mix of confidence, excitement, and fear. Being from Montana, she had not spent a lot of time on the ocean, but she had been inspired by the opportunity to challenge herself. Rylee was preparing to paddleboard from the Bahamas to Florida as part of an event called The Crossing for Cystic Fibrosis put on by *Piper's Angels Foundation*. "I remember sitting on the beach and being deathly afraid because you are looking out, you don't see any buildings, you don't see any lights," Rylee reflected. "You are going into the dark abyss. You have no idea what is coming your way."

As part of a team of four, Rylee paddled through the night and crossed 80 miles of ocean, battling sea sickness, fatigue, and self-doubt. When she hit the beach in Florida twelve hours later, she was overcome by emotions: "First thing I thought was, you just did this! I felt proud." Even after completing this amazing achievement with her team, Rylee felt a sense of incompletion. She knew she had more to give. She set her goal for the following year to do the 80 miles paddling solo. Unfortunately, as the paddlers assembled in the Bahamas in June 2024, weather forced postponement, and ultimately cancellation for those doing the full event. Undaunted, Rylee plans to continue her training so that she can make The Crossing solo in 2025.

When Rylee was training for The Crossing in 2023, she was taking Trikafta and felt that it had given her an extra boost of energy and health. Initially, she experienced a lot of side effects. She described, "That was such a down month. And I had no idea I was not happy. I was overwhelmed. My body was changing, and I was just not having it." Eventually, she was able to take it without the side effects, at least until a month before the 2024 Crossing. Her psychological issues once again returned and she faced the catch-22 of mental health versus physical health.[92] Rylee isn't sure if she will have to, or be able to, return to taking Trikafta. One thing is for sure, she will do everything she can to weather the storm of her Trikafta battle so she can cross the ocean solo on a paddleboard in June 2025.

The organization that puts on the epic oceanic event, *Piper's Angels Foundation*, was founded by executive director Travis Suit and is named after his daughter, Piper. Cystic fibrosis is very prevalent in Travis's family. His sister LeAnn was diagnosed at the age of forty when she became ill and had half of her lung removed. A year later, Travis's daughter Piper was diagnosed at the age of four,

---

92. The catch-22 was explained in chapter 7.

when she was sick with pneumonia. Following these diagnoses, Travis and his sister Nikki were also found to have CF, although with fewer manifestations than LeAnn and Piper. Witnessing the severity of CF's impact on his daughter, Travis sought to combine the salt water of the ocean with Piper's medications and treatments, to keep her as healthy as possible. He reflected, "It . . . was a gift to us for her health, and for her and [me], as a father and daughter, to do something and enjoy being out on the water together."[93]

Travis slowly learned to paddleboard and surf, which led to his idea to apply his newfound interest toward helping his daughter in another way. He explained, "I saw some paddleboarders out doing long-distance crossing between the islands [in Hawaii] and thought well, Florida and the Bahamas, the Gulf stream is going north; if we start paddling, eventually we will get there!" His inspiration became a reality in 2013. Connecting with the *CF Foundation,* it was called Crossing for a Cure. As Piper became sicker, Travis thought of other possible ways to help CF families: "That is when the impetus and the momentum to create an organization that focuses specifically on the needs of the patients and families arose." They rebranded The Crossing in 2017, now known as The Crossing for Cystic Fibrosis.

Piper's Angels provides numerous programs for families beyond The Crossing fundraiser. They have scholarships to help those with CF get equipment and training to be on the ocean, provide meals to those admitted to the hospital, and provide financial assistance. Travis explained, "So when a family needs it, to fix their car to keep going to the hospital . . . addressing urgent financial assistance . . . and seeing other needs that are arising, like mental health needs [we are there to help]." Attempting to meet the needs of families has led to the development of other programs, such as the mindfulness and meditation program, peer support groups, and their breath coaching program. Travis affirmed: "If you are going to help them live longer,

---

93. The ocean mist contains sodium chloride from the saltwater that acts as a "hypertonic" solution that promotes fluid to shift, leading to the thinning of mucus and hydrating the airways.

you got to help them live stronger. . . . If you are going to give people hope for a cure, you have to give them hope for today." His vision, along with the organization and its volunteers, have created remarkable awareness, financial assistance, and advocacy for those with CF to ameliorate the severity of the storm.

Casey McCullough, a former CF dietitian, is the director of operations and programs at *Piper's Angels Foundation*. When the clinic where she worked closed, *Piper's Angels* offered her a chance to continue to work with those with CF. Casey reflected, "I'm in a place of gratitude that everything has come full circle." Her role allows her to balance her enjoyment of helping those with CF, as well as introducing them to ocean sports. She is also a three-time world champion in skimboarding. Like Rylee, she has a goal for the next Crossing. Casey hopes to complete the entire 80 miles prone paddling, meaning she will be laying down on the paddleboard with only her arms to propel her on the journey. She continues to challenge herself, not only to raise funds for those with CF, but because she is inspired by the way those in the CF community continue to rise above the storm.

Tyler Engle has benefited from the largess of *Piper's Angels*. Seven years ago, he was in the hospital when he learned about Travis. The nurse asked him to write down a few snacks that he would like during his time at the hospital. Suddenly, Travis showed up with the snacks. A few years later, Tyler was in the hospital again, this time for four weeks with a PICC line. Travis, once again, brought some things to help him out. Tyler expressed, "The guy is absolutely amazing. The stuff he will do for total strangers is just crazy." Following that hospital stay, Tyler became interested in The Crossing. *Piper's Angels* was able to get him a paddleboard through one of their scholarships and he trained for a year for the 2023 Crossing. He said emotionally, "They are amazing people, for sure. They have . . . done more for me than my own family."

Tyler, who is twenty-eight years old, never expected to see thirty, much less be well enough to paddle across the ocean. Although healthy as a toddler, he became sicker as he grew up. "From sixteen to twenty-four, I'd spend four months a year in the hospital getting

IVs," he recalled. In March 2020, he took Trikafta. A few days later, following the purge, he woke up and didn't cough. He thought, "What is going on? What is happening?" He was shocked at the way his body was working. He emotionally shared, "It's pretty much like I don't have CF." During his frequent hospital stays, Tyler had begun to lose hope. Now, he can think about growing old and setting out to do things that seem impossible. He can cross the ocean on a paddleboard, buoyed by a community of care and a body that works as it was designed to work.

Ashley Williams has also benefited from the community of *Piper's Angels*. Her daughter Aurora was born with CF in 2020. She learned of Aurora's diagnosis early in the hospital. "You knew it was bad that the doctor sat down. It was like in one of the movies," she tearfully reflected. She was told that there were many things Aurora couldn't do, which was hard for her to handle. So far in her young life, Aurora has not been as sick as the doctors described. "Other than having a few operations at birth, she has been okay, but it has been a constant struggle to keep her well," explained Ashley.

When the doctors told her about Aurora's diagnosis, Ashley knew little about CF, other than the One Republic song, "I Lived." She began research to find CF organizations. Ashley has quickly grown to love the CF community and has tried to give back in any way she can. She has been involved in numerous fundraisers and is always trying to spread the word about the importance of advocacy and fundraising. Being involved in the CF community led her to *Piper's Angels*. Like Tyler, she was excited to participate in The Crossing in 2023, raising funds to help children like Aurora experience a better life.

The abyss of the ocean is an apt metaphor for the CF experience. Rylee offered, "I think of how unpredictable [CF] is and the ocean is unpredictable. . . . Anything can happen." Sometimes the ocean can squelch hope, especially when the waves become fierce. Despite the challenges, Emily Dickinson's "little bird" flies into "the storm" like the paddlers rowing into the waves. Sore must be the CF storm for many who fight each day to stay above the waves. Hope can arise out of the inspiration of doing the seemingly impossible and doing anything one can for the love of a child with an incurable disease. The bird of hope, with the aid of community, can strike out against the storm, daring the crossing of the ocean for Piper and many others.

The Little Bird

I recently asked my parents how they felt the day I was born. I knew I arrived six weeks early via an emergency C-section due to complications and that I was diagnosed with CF at birth. And they previously told me that another baby had been born with CF while I was in the hospital, and that the other child did not survive. My father recalled, "The doctor came out to talk to me and told me you had CF. I was surprised and said, 'Isn't that terminal?' The doctor responded 'Yes,' and walked away." I was in the NICU, in Cincinnati Children's Hospital, for three months. Doctors were constantly trying new things to keep me alive. My mother said, "We came every day to make sure you were okay." Eventually, they had a strong desire to bring me home, feeling the doctors had done all they could do to stabilize me. My mother emotionally told the doctors that she "just wanted to hold her son." She recalled, "After three months' time, I said to your dad that we have to get him home. We have to get him out of there."

When I came home from the hospital, my parents described how elated they were and praised the doctors for their care. They were also happy that I was not as sick as some of the other babies. All of this was a surprise for my parents, who did not expect to have a child. "I was just happy to have you. I was forty years old," my mother exclaimed with a giggle. They both optimistically reflected, "We never thought that you wouldn't live. We never gave up hope that you would make it."

I found talking to parents of young children who have CF to be a powerful window into loving someone with the disease. Just like my father, these parents described learning that their child was born with CF and all the uncertainty that comes with it. While I experienced the powerlessness of the human condition before suffering and death many times as a chaplain, it has never been connected to CF. Listening to the experiences of parents of children with CF affected me profoundly, as each touched a part of my own story, of my parents' hope and the sacrifice of caring for a young child with a chronic illness.

Doctors suspected Paula van Wyk's son Jack had CF shortly after his birth. Other members of Paula's family have CF, so she knew a little about the disease. Upon hearing Jack had CF, she hoped that his manifestation would be less severe, like her family. Unfortunately, that was not the case. At three months old, Jack began taking enzymes and has already been hospitalized, before the age of five. The number of treatments Jack requires each day is a challenge, especially when traveling. Their family recently traveled from their home in Canada to Mexico. Paula reflected, "My biggest concern was how am I going to get through the airport with all of his meds and equipment. I'm going to get stopped." The bag that was selected for search at the border was the bag with Jack's medications. Paula was afraid they would seize it, and they would have to leave the country immediately. Luckily, she could explain to the border agents and had doctors' notes for everything. Paula is still fearful when they travel: "By the time you get to your vacation spot your anxieties are so worked up. . . . It's going to take a while to actually enjoy your vacation."

Jack should be eligible for Trikafta when he is old enough under Canadian eligibility restrictions, which may mean traveling with less medications. "I never thought about the possibility of being able to travel with less medical equipment. I haven't been able to fathom that yet," Paula processed. More important than travel, of course, is the possibility that Jack may live a longer life. "I know people who have died [from CF], and I know people who have had lung transplants. It gave them a couple of years and then that was it. So, that . . . terrifies me," Paula said emotionally, when thinking about what might be in the future for Jack. "My biggest fear is I will have to bury my child."

Research and new technologies point to a brighter future for children like Jack than what would have been possible a short time ago. Paula expressed, "Things like Trikafta . . . that brings me hope I am not going to have to see him with ports and going through lung transplants." Medical advancements give Paula hope that she won't have to bury Jack, just as my own experience with Trikafta gives me hope that my parents won't have to bury me. These possibilities are a profound gift, and a privilege. Looking to the future with hope for what could be, rather than focusing on the despair of the present, are the wings that carry the CF community into the future. This is especially true for parents who would do anything to give their child a chance at a more "normal" life.

Collette Portner knows this hope as well. Her daughter Ravyn is eight years old. When Ravyn was born, Collette was told by doctors what to expect having a child with CF, but she reflects, "nothing that they told me is anything like what it is now." This is partly because of gene modulators and partly because Ravyn's CF manifestation has been fairly healthy. Since starting Trikafta, Ravyn has not been hospitalized with lung issues. Collette reflected, "Now she fights colds, which is crazy, better than anyone in our house." So far, Trikafta has helped keep CF "on the back burner," allowing Ravyn to do most things like other children. Ravyn still does her daily treatments. "Having a child with cystic fibrosis is not the easiest thing … it's hard sometimes to get kids to do stuff they don't want to do," she reflected, echoing the sentiments of many CF parents.

Although Collette was clearly grateful for Ravyn's progress, she expressed that she is not blind to reality: "I have that hope, but at the same time, I'm realistic, anything can happen, you know, at any time." She doesn't want to set herself up for sadness because the long-term effects of Trikafta are unknown. "It becomes more of a gamble as people with cystic fibrosis get older. . . . These medicines are amazing, but you don't know at the end of the day," she acknowledged. For now, Ravyn is thriving and Collette is grateful that her daughter has a possible future. Echoing the same desire as Paula did for Jack, Collette emotionally added, "I'm hopeful. . . . I just hope she outlives me." Love and hope go hand in hand as these parents hope their children live long enough to grow up.

While Jack and Ravyn are too young to understand the reality of having CF, Maeve, the daughter of Liz Hammel, is a recent college graduate beginning her adult life. Maeve grew up in Vermont and was diagnosed with CF at the age of two. "It was a big shock and a learning curve," Liz described. Growing up, Maeve was in and out of the hospital with lung exacerbations, despite being very compliant with her treatments. "She never resisted doing any of the therapies…I guess we kind of fit them into all the things we would normally do," Liz explained.

In early 2020, Maeve began taking Trikafta. She is now maintaining a healthy weight and is recovering from illness much faster. Perhaps the most exciting change has been the removal of her port following a CT scan that revealed her lungs were looking better with no progression of deterioration. Liz explained, "That…made us believe that Trikafta has really changed things in significant ways." Symbolic of this transformation is that Maeve was able to study abroad in Spain for five months. Liz said emotionally, "I realized that I've only been worried about the things that everybody worries about when their kids go abroad." As Maeve leaves the metaphorical nest to find her own way as an adult, she does so with new hope and possibilities. When the time comes, hopefully Jack and Ravyn will have the same chances, to enter the world without CF restrictions. This hope is exemplified in the stories of parents doing everything they can with the hope that their children can outlive them.

Pat Mitchell has hope as well. Her hope is for her great-grandson, Hudson Parker. Both Pat and Hudson have CF. Pat is seventy-nine years old, and Hudson is three. "I want to be there for his college graduation," Pat said tenderly. She has lived most of her life in New York and was born the twelfth of thirteen children. Two of her siblings also have CF. Her diagnosis came late in life at the age of sixty, unlike Hudson, who was diagnosed at birth due to pancreatic and other health complications. Despite these challenges, Pat explained that Hudson always seems to be happy. "He is so cute, I love being with him," she gushed. Trikafta has been a huge help for Pat and came at a time when her health was declining quickly. She hopes that Hudson will have the same experience with

Trikafta. "This hope is that there is a future for him," described a great-grandmother whose heart is full of hope and love.

One of my earliest childhood memories is my mother reading *Are You My Mother?*, a book by PD Eastman. The story is about a baby bird who falls out of his nest when the mother goes to get him worms. The bird travels to many animals asking each if she is his mother. I remember feelings of fear and worry coming over me when the bird could not find his mother. At the end of the story, a large machine places the bird back in the nest just as his mother returns. I remember the relief I felt when the baby bird and his mother reunited. Perhaps, as my mother read, she reflected on the months I was in the NICU as she pleaded to "just hold her son." That baby bird was looking for the thing with feathers, never giving up hope. A lesson of love and determination for us all.

Chapter 12

Paying Attention

Having CF makes me different. In some ways, this means there are things I can't do, and I have grown to accept that limitation. On the other hand, I have a unique way of seeing the world. I think when people are sick, they can realize a lot about the meaning of life. I know I would not be the person I am if I had been born without cystic fibrosis. I hope there is a way I can share that perspective, that wisdom, with the world. I must remember to boldly be myself because there is only one of me for all time. Goodnight.

Living with a chronic illness can offer a person a unique perspective. Living within CF Time, CF Space, and CF World are experiences for those who live with a daily struggle or who are coming to terms with life in their advanced years. During each interview of someone living with CF, I asked them what wisdom they gained from having CF. Some spoke of ways that CF gave them perspectives on navigating the external world, while others looked inward to see how it formed them as individuals. The wisdom offered was a beautiful exposition of how suffering and tragedy can give perspective and insight. When the roses speak, one can gain wisdom by paying attention.

Reframing Perspective

As a hospital chaplain, I learned a lot from my patients. While I served as their chaplain, they served as my teachers about the fragility of

209

life, the beauty of relationships, and the importance of living fully. One morning I met with a woman in her late eighties for a pre-op prayer. Usually, these are short visits before surgery. In this case, the patient and her daughter had arrived a bit early, so I was able to spend more time with them. While the procedure was not imminently life-threatening, any surgery for a person in her late eighties carries a heightened risk. She spoke about moving from her home to live with her daughter and then shared a story about a deer in her yard and how she watched the mother deer care for her fawns. Through these stories, I began to see a theme of care for others emerging. I eventually asked her how it feels to be the one *needing* care. Her eyes appeared tearful as she acknowledged it was hard for her to move in with her daughter and that she did not want to be a burden. Her daughter emotionally assured her that she was welcome.

This conversation may have been a breakthrough for this mother and daughter, where the mother was able to voice her vulnerability, and her daughter was able to affirm her love. The beauty of this tender moment stuck with me as well. It was moments like that that affirmed my desire to move closer to Cincinnati to be with my parents, whose age was close to this woman's age. The importance of caring for my parents was one of my biggest insights from chaplaincy. I had never thought about seeing my parents grow old because I always expected to die first. Just as this family was able to see their relationship dynamics differently, I was able to see my relationship with my parents in a new way through the tenderness of this woman and her daughter. This visit was a gift for us both.

Another way to look at this concept is the term "reframing." A number of years ago, a friend offered this as a way for me to get through a difficult time. She encouraged me to step outside the difficulty as much as possible and to examine it from multiple perspectives. That does not mean diminishing a difficulty by saying it could always be worse. Such "advice" can often be used to minimize the pain or experience of another and can do more harm than good. Reframing is seeing the greater context of a situation. When this transformation comes from within, rather than by being imposed from outside, it may mitigate a difficult circumstance.

"With every broken bone, I swear I lived," sings One Republic in the song "I Lived." While this song has special significance to Brynn Baskin, Ashley Williams, and many of us in the CF community, it is especially meaningful to Bryan Warnecke. Bryan was a teenager when he was offered the chance to be the person with CF in the official music video. He and his father had participated in a biking fundraiser where they rode over 1000 miles in forty-three days and raised $300,000 for CF research. His hospital recommended him when One Republic was looking for someone in the CF community who had an amazing story to tell. Bryan reflected, "It was a pretty incredible experience. Red Rocks, where it is filmed, is my second home."

In light of the video and his CF experience, Bryan offered, "What you are going through isn't permanent. . . . No matter how messed up we are, all you have to do is change your perspective ten degrees and you can see the world in a whole new light." This form of reframing has given him strength during many difficult times. "I Lived" has been especially helpful and Bryan thinks of it as "the fuel to keep my fire burning" when he encounters difficulty. He strives to live and enjoy life as much as possible. "I never let CF slow me down," he affirmed. Whether it is another long-distance bike ride, exploring the mountainside, or spending time with loved ones, he wants to make sure that when his time comes, he will look back and say, "I lived."

Reframing can also be described as putting daily difficulties into perspective. Clark Thiemann lives in Connecticut and has had tremendous results from Trikafta: "Thirty-six hours after taking it there was something different about how I felt. It was pretty magical," he recollected. The medication will allow him to spend more years with his two daughters and his wife than he would have thought possible when his daughters were born. He also explained, "The quality of life that doesn't show up on tests is the flexibility that you can go away for the weekend and not have to carry 200 pounds worth of stuff to keep yourself feeling okay." The wisdom of having CF has made Clark "less 'me' focused and less worried about the gravity of the small things that you have to deal with every day." He rarely gets worked up over the "little things" and he is better able to focus on "things that really matter." When you live with a chronic illness, it helps to put things into perspective, and Clark is grateful that CF has taught him to better distinguish the major challenges versus the bumps in the road.

Erica Daley expressed a similar sentiment. She did not find out she had CF until her fifties. Although she had some medical issues along the way, she was healthy enough that doctors did not test her for CF until she was in the emergency room coughing up blood. "I thought I was dying. It was a really bad time for me," she reflected. "Once [it] developed," she explained, "it was full CF; it just took time to get there in my timeline of life." She expressed the wisdom that having CF taught her as "You can't tell people how to feel, you feel the way you feel." Navigating so many difficulties in life has made Erica a more resilient person: "Focus on the things you can control and not on the things you can't control." She described that you may not be able to control that you have a chronic disease, but "you can control what you do with the time you have." A powerful message from someone who found out later in life that she has an incurable illness. "Life is short. . . . Don't let CF win, and keep fighting," she emphatically shared.

Helen Roper's wisdom has similarities to Clark's and Erica's. She reflected, "You see people getting upset about stupid, small things and you think, does it really matter?" CF helps Helen put experiences into perspective. She lives in the UK and was on the transplant list for three years before Trikafta stabilized her lung function. She recalled the day after she took Trikafta, "I remember waking and my lungs are amazing, full of moisture. . . . It felt like they'd been to the spa and they'd had a massage." Her lung function remains around 40% and her health still prevents her from working, but that hasn't stopped Helen from experiencing life and appreciating the time she has left. "I am very much of the mindset of make hay while the sun shines and appreciate what we can," she said thoughtfully. Her wisdom is born from her experiences in life and surviving the challenges of having a chronic illness:

"You learn to be patient and take the good days as they come . . . and enjoy things as much as possible," Helen shared.

Everyone Has a Broken Heart

Working toward positivity and removing self-doubt are ways of reframing and ways of caring for oneself. Sometimes positivity can help a person remain healthy in the face of difficult challenges and a difficult prognosis. At times, feeling sad and hopeless may cause one's body to become weaker and a person to wear down more. It can be hard to maintain a positive outlook in the face of suffering and loss, especially when the boulder of CF Space appears to be heaviest. That does not mean every circumstance has a silver lining. Sometimes things are bad, suffering is great, and death is close. There are also times when a positive mindset can have transformative changes.

Dugan Reilly lives in Nashville, Tennessee, and has worked to transform his mindset and the mindset of others. Growing up with CF, he realized he was different from other people: "You really start to get used to it [the hospital], it is like your second home." CF taught him the importance of taking time to know who you are on the inside and what that may mean for a career. Dugan explained, "If you really want to figure out what to do, think of your interests. What are those areas you would like to look at and explore?" He has translated these insights into helping others, especially the chronically ill. His goal in working with others is to "help them with their mindset and really break out of negative thoughts." Dugan has learned these skills from his own vocational journey. He realized that working a typical day job would be difficult given his medical condition; so, he adapted. "I saw real estate as a way of making great money but also having control of my time and being able to do what I want, when I can do it," he explained. Coming to know oneself and the way an illness or condition can affect current realities and future possibilities is a question that those with a chronic illness are always asking themselves; finding people to help explore those questions can be helpful.

"I'm always trying to see things in a positive way, as daft as it can be. . . . Just take one thing at a time," expressed Justyna Zaskwara, echoing similar perspectives as Dugan. This is a powerful statement for a woman who was told her chance of surviving when she was born in Poland was small: "The doc didn't really give much hope . . . because I had been too poorly and was full of chest infections." She currently lives in the UK and has seen some improvement in her health with Trikafta. "It is just opening a lot of doors," she explained of her new opportunities. She still gets sick and can struggle to remain positive with the rollercoaster of her health. Dealing with lung infections and COVID have reminded Justyna that despite having positive results with Trikafta, CF will always be part of her life. Living on the rollercoaster is a constant reminder of the need to take things one day at a time and in the most positive way possible.

A positive mindset may mean doing the daily activities that are required for good health. Anissa Hostetter knows the importance of taking care of herself. She lives in Ohio and was born in 1970. Upon returning from a trip to Maui in 2016, she ended up in the ICU coughing up blood. She recalled, "I was put into a medically induced coma because my lung collapsed. They didn't think I was going to live." Over time she recovered and attended rehab to regain her strength. She is currently taking Trikafta and has not seen much difference in her PFT. She does have a bit more strength and reflected, "My husband is a fast walker and now I can keep up with him. So, I am able to walk a little quicker without getting winded." Anissa offered some wisdom that has enabled her to live into her fifties with CF: "You have to take care of yourself. I don't remember ever going through a time when I didn't want to do therapy, treatments, or pills." She also credits the care of her parents, and a bit of luck. While some people may not have gone to the hospital following a vacation, Anissa knew she had to go, and likely survived because of it. The more people inhabit CF Space and feel the weight of the boulder of treatments, the harder it can be to keep doing what needs to be done. Anissa's reflection is a good reminder that self-care and adherence are ways of reframing the potential hopelessness of living with a chronic illness.

Teresa Dunning also reflected on the importance of self-care. She had respiratory problems for much of her life and was diagnosed with CF in her sixties. Prior to Trikafta, she found it difficult to do anything because of her breathing: "I couldn't go upstairs, I couldn't go for a walk, it just took so much out of me. . . . If I [had not] started the CF medicine I wouldn't be here today." When she visited her CF clinic in New York, they were amazed at the transformation of her breathing. Teresa also credits her self-care toward still being alive today. Her husband sells firewood; helping him and remaining active have been very helpful for her. She explained, "Exercise is a big thing. . . . By doing the exercise, it really helped me a lot as far as regaining my strength and my breathing." Having almost died twice from CF has not only affirmed the importance of her self-care but has given her an appreciation for the time she has left.

Having a chronic illness can also be transformative for how you treat other people. Paula van Wyk's mother once told her, "Treat everybody like they have a broken heart because you don't know what someone is going through by looking at them."[94] Caring for Jack has brought home this wisdom even more. "CF is an invisible illness," Paula reflected, explaining how one can look at Jack and many people with CF and not think they are dealing with a serious medical condition. By assuming everyone is dealing with something, that everyone carries a burden, it leads to giving people the benefit of the doubt, rather than stern judgment. No one knows what it is like to be someone else, and no one lives a life free of pain. At some point everyone may experience a broken heart.

McKenzie Schneider expects to be able to live out Paula's mom's advice in her future vocation. She believes that having CF gives her a "sense of independence and responsibility." She explained, "Starting from an early age, you learn how to take your medications, do treatments, and you learn more about your health in general." She

---

94. Paula's experience as a mother to Jack, who has CF, was discussed in chapter 11.

acknowledged it was hard, mentally and physically, when she began college. Once she figured out how to balance her medical treatments, the sense of responsibility helped give her the balance to succeed. She recently graduated from the University of Montana Pharmacy School, a vocational pursuit that grew from her CF experience. "I feel like I'm able to relate to a lot of the patients, too, as far as their hardships with diseases," she reflected. When ill patients come to have their prescriptions filled, McKenzie will be able to express empathy with them because she knows the struggle of being ill. People with a chronic condition usually have to grow up a bit faster than their peers and sometimes this results in a drive to succeed.

During the first day of my CPE internship, we watched a video entitled *Empathy: The Human Connection to Patient Care*.[95] Our educators told us, "You will see these people every day." The video depicts various "invisible" realities that people inhabit as they move through the Cleveland Clinic: a family going to see a loved one for the last time, a person waiting for an organ, an elderly couple who do not understand what their doctor is explaining, and numerous others. One scene is of a mother hoping to hold her baby for the first time, which I immediately connected to my own mother's desire to hold me. I thought of this often, realizing that each person at the hospital has a story. Eventually, my realization expanded to people I saw outside the hospital. It is true. I see these people every day. One does not need to be in a hospital to carry a story of a broken heart or to recognize others who are carrying their own.

Molly Jensen shared a story that combines some of the wisdom of internal transformation and encountering others with love.[96] When she was fourteen, Molly was in the hospital for IVs and was placed on the cancer patient floor because there were no open rooms on the CF floor. "As I walked past rooms," she recalled, "I realized that their circumstances were so much sadder than mine." She saw children who were too sick to get up and walk, and some

95. Cleveland Clinic, *Empathy: The Human Connection*, https://www.youtube.com/watch?v=cDDWvj_q-o8.
96. Molly's experience with CF Time was shared in chapter 1.

who were crying: "I sat in my bed that night and I cried too." She thought about how lucky she was that she was able to walk, and her attitude about being in the hospital changed. She decided to do something nice for the kids on the floor. With the help of the nurses and her mother, she made paper turkeys for Thanksgiving and wrote messages on them. While making them, her mindset changed from feeling sorry for herself for being in the hospital to wanting to help those who were struggling. She found that in giving to others she was also helping herself: "It changed my perspective from 'I hate being here' . . . to 'I'm healthy enough that I can make things.'" She knows this isn't easy, especially when things are bad. But sometimes reframing your experience and remembering that everyone has a broken heart can make an important difference.

Conclusion

Garden Seeds

Roses grow from seeds. Seeds do not develop into roses overnight. Like most things of beauty, it takes time and nurturing to create a flower. For some, nurturing involves the belief that there is an order to the universe, encapsulated in a God of power and love. For others, nurturing is about honoring those who have been lost and sacrificing so that the young have a future. Wisdom offers a way to share the insights of a life well lived so that others may grow from that knowledge. Part Four brings to a close this journey through the rose garden by sitting with universal questions that all human beings may share—the beyond in our midst and living a life of hope. The roses who have spoken through this book are unique in many ways; still, they ask similar questions. What does it mean to be alive? What does it mean to plant seeds for the time when we are no longer alive?

Lyndall Grace hopes to help plant seeds for teenagers who, like her, have CF. In the past few years, she has become a well-known CF advocate, especially in her home country of Australia. Lyndall recalls finding out that she was living in CF Time when she googled CF as a teenager and learned her life expectancy: "I think at that point it really changed how I would look at my life or my career prospects, [and] my relationship prospects, because I might not make it to thirty." After high school, she began to get sick and she became allergic to some of the medications used to fight her infections, which caused more declines: "After that, I managed to get off of the steroids. I didn't go back to the clinic for three years, which was a lot. I had a very bad relationship with CF."

Her health rollercoaster eventually settled down into a slow decline, but these early years of struggling with adhering to her treatments had a profound impact on the type of work she hoped to do in the future. She explained,

> When I was a teenager, I wanted absolutely nothing to do with any of it. And I feel like that's where . . . teenagers drop off is when they don't want to be any different. So, they stopped listening to their doctors; they stopped going to their appointments; they fight their parents all the time because they just don't want to be different. And I know that's how I felt because I didn't have any friends with CF. . . . I think it is also that time when you get slapped in the face with your mortality when you are a teenager; and then I feel like you go through this massive, crazy point in your life. . . . Your hormones are all over the place and you're dealing with the idea of mortality at fifteen. . . . Having other teenagers talk to teenagers about it and connecting that community rather than them just going off in an isolated fashion and being like, I want nothing to do with this [is an area I would like to explore].

Lyndall's voice in CF advocacy blossomed when she appeared on *Married at First Sight Australia*. She applied to be on the show because she had recently begun taking Trikafta and thought, "I was in this euphoria of gratefulness and excitement for my life. I essentially applied because I was like, I can get married, I can have kids, I can do these things now!" She went into the show open to finding the love of her life. She also went in knowing it would be a national platform for CF. Although she did not end up staying with her partner from the show, she found something even more meaningful. She explained that in making her final decision to not remain with her co-star, "If there is one thing CF has given me, it is resilience. For the first time in my life, I am able to give my unwavering commitment to somebody. I have lived so restricted in many areas of my life, but now I will not be restricted by my condition. I will not be restricted by my body. I will not be restricted by my fear." Lyndall wants to help others feel the same way, especially teenagers who may think they are nothing more than the disease they carry. She wants to help others, especially those who have been pigeonholed by a medical condition, to find their voice and their self-worth, just as she did when she was able to make her relationship choice. Lyndall wants to plant seeds in the rose garden so that others can discover themselves. One doesn't need to be a celebrity to embark upon the same mission as Lyndall. One just needs to be true to one's character and to have a vision of helping other roses bloom.

Afterword

Whirl Is King

In March 1996, I was given a glimpse into a possible future when I opened a school newspaper and read a headline. I saw that the trajectory of my disease would likely require a lung transplant in my late twenties. I unknowingly learned a valuable life lesson—that "we have time" is the greatest lie ever told. On January 1, 2020, Trikafta diverted me onto a new path and has extended my life. However, I will still die. As I tell my students, "We all die. But not all of us truly live." The delicate balance of knowing one will die and trying to decide what that means for life is an ongoing journey. Those who live each day with a chronic illness are some of the best teachers for discerning how to proceed on that pilgrimage. I often wonder what to do with my new lease on life, while I also know that the ground upon which this lease rests could shift at any time.

Darren Turner, who lives in California, lives his life to the fullest and challenges himself by climbing mountains. He described his experience with CF as being "generally pretty healthy." Taking Trikafta has resulted in a bit more energy and less coughing. Darren's health has enabled him to explore his love of hiking. A month after the pandemic began, he and a few friends got a permit to climb Mt. Whitney, the tallest point in the contiguous United States. Darren slowly worked up to it and in July 2020, they ascended Mt. Whitney in two days. He reflected, "Sometimes when I go up [Interstate] 395, I'll stop to look at it. I actually did that! I got all the way up there. It's still . . . hard to believe." Darren conquered 14,505 feet of mountain. He doesn't let chronic illness define what he can do in life. He challenges the stereotypes and ascends to the heights. While I won't climb Mt. Whitney, Darren's story gives me hope and inspiration to find my next "mountain," the place where people with CF are told they can never ascend.

Adrian Flor uses his legs for a different purpose than Darren. He doesn't ascend mountains; he runs great distances. Adrian lives in Australia and describes his CF manifestation as "quite fortunate." He is married, has two children, and is thirty-nine years old. Only once has he been hospitalized for CF-related illness. Before taking Trikafta, his lung function was 101%. Now it is 113%. Adrian explained, "My lung function has been preserved, not only . . . from Trikafta, but from running. The running has . . . kept it [at] about the 100% mark." Like Darren, he thinks Trikafta has helped open up even more possibilities of what he can achieve. He ran the Sydney Marathon on September 17, 2023, and achieved this feat in four hours and twenty minutes. He runs not only for his health but to demonstrate to his kids that hard work and dedication can pay off. While I can no longer run marathons, Adrian's story gives me hope and inspiration to find my next "race," the place where people with CF are told they can never keep up.

A new lease on life has helped Erika Castrucci imagine dancing with her son at his wedding. Erika lives in Canada and began her Trikafta journey on December 24, 2021. She described it as "The best Christmas gift the world has ever given me." Although she experienced a rash when she initially took it, this side effect paled in comparison to the transformation of her health. Her PFT increased from 67% to 103%. At seeing this result, she recalled, "I cried in disbelief. To go from knocking on death's door to breathing as some-one unaffected by cystic fibrosis in less than a month is astounding to me." Although she still does her daily treatments, Trikafta has given her the chance "to realistically dream of growing old with my husband." While I do not have a spouse or children, Erika's story gives me hope that I will be able to grow old with those I love and treasure those moments like a Christmas gift I never expected.[97]

---

97. In lieu of an interview, Erika sent me a reflection she wrote, part of which can be found here: https://www.cysticfibrosis.ca/blog/erikas-story/.

Kathleen Schwartz's challenge comes from her vocational desires. After high school, she attended a community college and took courses to prepare to be a nurse. These aspirations were not completely supported by her doctors who worried that having CF could cause her to get sick working in the hospital. In 2018, she worked for nine months as a Certified Nursing Assistant (CNA) and was always sick. She decided to change course, a decision that was "the worst breakup I have ever had. Deciding not to go into nursing . . . sucked . . . because I know that is what I am good at." She decided to complete a degree in health administration. When her younger sister graduated from a nurse practitioner program, Kathleen was happy for her, but she was reminded of what she had to walk away from. "It literally broke my heart. . . . That was supposed to be me," she said emotionally.

Trikafta has given Kathleen the chance she never expected. "With Trikafta, I decided I am going to go to nursing school. It is something I don't feel like I have to give up anymore," she said confidently. Her new lease on life may lead her to become a nurse who will use her kindness and sense of humor to put people at ease when they are going through difficult times. Kathleen explained, "It [Trikafta] has given me a new life that I want, and I am excited for it now. I get to do what I want." While I will not become a nurse, Kathleen's story gives me hope and inspiration to find my next "destination," the place where people with CF are told they do not belong.

The "destination" of hospital chaplaincy is one of those places where people with CF would rarely venture for fear of getting sick, especially before Trikafta. The final visit of my chaplain residency was a call to the bedside of a woman in a coma. She was near my age and had suffered an unexpected episode. As I walked to the elevator, I thought of the similarities to my first solo internship visit. I thought of my previous anxiety and fear and how much I had learned in fifteen months. Upon arrival, I invited the family together and we prayed in a circle around her. I then remained to comfort the family over this tragedy, inviting them to share a bit about her life. Fifteen months earlier, I hid in the back of a hospital room and left the room feeling fear. Now, I was serving as a chaplain, sitting with the patient's teenage son during the worst day of his life. This visit revealed to me how much I had grown. Like Darren, I had ascended a mountain that I never thought possible. I had not only crossed a threshold to a place where people with CF rarely go; I had crossed a threshold in my own growth in self-awareness and confidence.

While many individuals have been able to achieve the previously unthinkable through gene modulators, the unity of the CF community has suffered from the diversification of possibilities. On my first day of college at John Carroll University, Dr. Dean Birch walked into our classroom and wrote on the board, "Whirl is king, having deposed Zeus." He pointed to the board and declared, "By the end of this term, you will understand what this means." This memory returned to me, as I reflected on the CF community in the era of gene modulators. Zeus, representing a single narrative, symbolizes a time when the CF community was united by similar circumstances. Now that so many are being aided by the miraculous results of gene modulators, whirl, or individual meta-narratives, is truly king. I realize I have allowed my transformation to cloud my realization that some with CF are still suffering, just as I was before Trikafta. The fight for a CF cure is not over. As I learned in chaplaincy, illness and loss can affect anyone at any time. Control is an illusion.

As I complete this book, I have returned to the place where this journey began. I have become like Mr. Luedeke, but in a way different from what I expected. I am now the teacher at St. Xavier who has cystic fibrosis, who can impact a student with a chronic illness, as Mr. Luedeke impacted me. Each time I stand in front of students, I carry his legacy with me. For now, my new lease on life will be spent in the classroom and will include advocacy for continued research for a cure. In this time where whirl is king, I will do my part to help those who have been left out of the gene modulator lifeboat. To do this, I will need to continue to grow in courage and confidence as I did during chaplaincy. Death is the one experience that awaits us all. Until then, I will draw inspiration from Robert Herrick's poem, gathering rosebuds while I can, as this same *rose* that smiles today, tomorrow will be dying. When eventually my petals drop foil by foil to the ground, I want to be able to look back at my life and sing from the depths of my fibrosed lungs, "I lived!"

Referenced Cystic Fibrosis Organizations

The author encourages you to learn more about these organizations dedicated to helping those with cystic fibrosis and their families.

The Bonnell Foundation
https://thebonnellfoundation.org

Boomer Esiason Foundation
https://www.esiason.org

CF Vests Worldwide
https://www.cfvww.org

Claire's Place Foundation
https://clairesplacefoundation.org

Cystic Fibrosis Australia
https://www.cysticfibrosis.org.au

Cystic Fibrosis Foundation (Canada)
https://www.cysticfibrosis.ca

Cystic Fibrosis Foundation (USA)
https://www.cff.org

Cystic Fibrosis Trust (UK)
https://www.cysticfibrosis.org.uk

Emily's Entourage
https://www.emilysentourage.org

The Jeffrey Palma Foundation, DBA Jeffrey's House
https://www.jeffreys-house.org

Piper's Angels Foundation
https://www.pipersangels.org

Rock CF Foundation
https://letsrockcf.org

Wish for Wendy Foundation
https://www.wishforwendy.org

Glossary

airway: System that allows oxygen to enter the bloodstream to nourish the body. This pathway includes your trachea that ends in a bifurcation (splits two ways) leading to the left and right main—or primary—bronchi. From the main bronchus, there is continuing division into smaller structures, with the progressive order being the lobar bronchi, followed by segmental bronchi, then bronchioles, and finally the alveoli (where the oxygen enters, and carbon dioxide exits the bloodstream).

AMS: Altered mental status refers to a change or any deviation in a person's cognitive functioning, behavior, or consciousness from their baseline or usual state; often a result of a broader issue (e.g., illness, toxins or imbalance, injuries, etc.).

B. cepacia: Bacteria found in the natural environment and not seen as a risk to *healthy* people. It is correlated with an increased decline in lung function in people with CF. Burkholderia bacteria tend to be resistant to many antibiotics.

bronchomalacia: Weakening of the cartilage in the wall(s) of the bronchial tube(s) that can easily collapse while breathing (during inhalation and/or exhalation) and can cause difficulty breathing, chronic cough, wheezing, increased difficulty clearing mucous, increased lung infections, and/or hypoxia (low oxygen levels in the blood). Chronic inflammation and damage to the airway from the presence of thick mucus in people with CF can weaken the bronchial cartilage. This is often referred to as *airway remodeling*—when the structure of the airway is changed.

CFTR: Cystic fibrosis transmembrane conductance regulator. People who genetically inherit two copies of a mutated CFTR gene will have cystic fibrosis.

CMO: Comfort measures only is a plan of care that directs efforts toward quality and comfort rather than focusing on treatment of the underlying condition.

compassionate use: This is also referred to as "expanded access" and is when a medication or vaccine is made accessible to those with a need deemed critical. These patients would not otherwise meet the eligibility criteria for approval.

CPE: Clinical pastoral education is interfaith professional education for clergy, ministers, and spiritual leaders that teaches spiritual care in a clinical setting. It meets the educational requirement for professional chaplain board certification.

FEV1: The forced expiratory volume (how much air you expel) in one second is the primary value referenced by patients with CF. This is measured through a pulmonary function test (PFT).

gene modulator therapy: Treatment that temporarily alters the genetic function of a gene. For those with cystic fibrosis, CFTR modulator therapies offer to correct/improve the function of the malfunctioning protein made by the mutated CFTR gene for the duration of the medication in their system.

hemoptysis: Coughing up blood, a common progression of CF due to infection and/or irritation of the pulmonary blood vessels that can cause them to become more delicate over time.

PICC line: A peripherally inserted central catheter line often inserted in the arm and advanced to a large central vein near the heart. It is used for long-term IV antibiotic medications.

PFT: A pulmonary function test provides physical measurements along with a *percent predicted* based on the average expectation for a healthy person of similar age, weight, and gender.

pseudomonas: A common pathogen in the lungs of people with CF that can be difficult to treat and becomes resistant to antibiotics. It can also cause infection and inflammation leading to further progression in the disease and a decline in lung function over time.

sweat test: A test performed using a technique to collect and measure the concentration of chloride in one's sweat. It is one way to diagnose CF. People with CF sweat higher levels of chloride (one of two components that make up sodium chloride or NaCl).

Bibliography

Amend, Andy. "Luedeke Battles CF." *Blueprint*. March 1, 1996.

Anderson, Carol. *White Rage*. Bloomsbury Publishing, 2016.

Carson, David, dir. *Star Trek: Generations*. Paramount Pictures, 1994.

Castrucci, Erika. "Erika's Story." *Cystic Fibrosis Canada*. July 8, 2022. https://www.cysticfibrosis.ca/blog/erikas-story/.

Cleveland Clinic. "Empathy: The Human Connection," https://www.youtube.com/watch?v=cDDWvj_q-o8.

Cystic Fibrosis Foundation. "About Cystic Fibrosis." https://www.cff.org/intro-cf/about-cystic-fibrosis.

Cystic Fibrosis Foundation. "65 Roses Story." https://www.cff.org/about-us/65-roses-story.

Cystic Fibrosis Foundation. "Types of CF Mutations." https://www.cff.org/research-clinical-trials/types-cftr-mutations#:~:text=There%20are%20five%20classes%20of,different%20types%20of%20CFTR%20mutations.

Day, Dorothy. *The Long Loneliness*. HarperCollins, 1952.

Espenhahn, Svenja. "Advocating for Access to Orphan Drugs: Beth and Madison Vanstone's Story." *Canadian Rare Disease Network*. May 14, 2022. https://canadianrdn.ca/advocating-for-access-to-orphan-drugs-beth-and-madison-vanstones-story/

Gamble, Vanessa Northington. "Under the Shadow of Tuskegee: African Americans and Healthcare." *American Journal of Public Health*. 87:11, November 1997.

Hanh, Thich Nhat. *Being Peace*. Parallax Press, 1987.

Heller, Joseph. *Catch-22*. Simon & Schuster, 1955.

Heo, Suyeon, David C. Young, Julie Safirstein, Brian Bourque, Martine Antell, Stefanie Diloreto, and Shannon Rotolo. "Mental status changes during elexacaftor/tezacaftor/ivacaftor therapy." *Journal of Cystic Fibrosis*. October 2021.

Koloroutis, Mary, and Michael Trout. *See Me as a Person: Creating Therapeutic Relationships*. Creative Healthcare Management, 2012.

Kurtz, Ernest, and Katherine Ketcham. *The Spirituality of Imperfection: Storytelling and the Search for Meaning*. Bantam Books, 1993.

Kushner, Harold S. *When Bad Things Happen to Good People*. Avon Books, 1981.

Lamas, Daniela J. "What It's Like to Learn You're Going to Live Longer than You Expected." *New York Times*. February 6, 2023. https://www.nytimes.com/2023/02/06/opinion/cystic-fibrosis-treatment.html

Lay, Kat. "South Africans take on big pharma for access to 'miracle' cystic fibrosis drug." *The Guardian*. March 18, 2024. https://www.theguardian.com/global-development/2024/mar/18/cystic-fibrosis-patient-south-africa-cheri-nel-lawsuit-big-pharma-generic-drugs-trikafta-access-vertex

Leader, Anton, dir. *The Twilight Zone*. "The Midnight Sun." November 1961.

Menkhaus, James. *Immersion: A Pilgrimage into Service*. New City Press, 2022.

Menkhaus, Jimmy. "The Eternal Spring." *With Every Breath*. Edited by Katherine Russell. Merrill Press, 2006.

Merton, Thomas. "Things in their Identity." In *Seeds of Contemplation*. New Directions, 1949.

Mueller, Rebecca. "The Genome and the Biome: Cystic Fibrosis @ 6 Feet Apart." Unpublished Dissertation, University of Pennsylvania, 2021.

National Heart, Lung, and Blood Institute (NIH). "Cystic Fibrosis Causes." https://www.nhlbi.nih.gov/health/cystic-fibrosis/causes#:~:text=Cystic%20fibrosis%20is%20an%20inherited,parent)%20will%20have%20cystic%20fibrosis.

Oord, Thomas Jay. *God Can't: How to Believe in God and Love after Tragedy, Abuse and Other Evils*. Sacra-Sage Press, 2019.

Sawtell-Rickson, Jye. "Quantifying the Thai Cave Rescue." *Medium*. September 28, 2018. https://jyesr.medium.com/the-thai-cave-rescue-248c5b08cbf0.

Shields, Michele, Allison Kastenbaum, and Laura B. Dunn. "Spiritual AIM and the Work of the Chaplain: A Model for Assessing Spiritual Needs and the Outcomes in Relationships." *Palliative Support Care*. 13:1 (2015).

Smith, Houston. *The World's Religions.* HarperCollins Publishers, 1991.

Smith, Martin. *The Football Boy Wonder: The Charlie Fry Series.* Create Space Publishing Platform, 2015.

Smith, Tita. "Why this brave Aussie woman is forced to fork out $21,375 a MONTH just to survive after doctors warned she had six months to live—but she's running out of money fast," in *Daily Mail Australia.* February 22, 2022. https://www.dailymail.co.uk/news/article-10538711/Aussie-woman-living-cystic-fibrosis-forced-fork-21-375-MONTH-just-survive.html.

Trivedi, Bijal. *Breath from Salt: A Deadly Genetic Disease, a New Era in Science, and the Patients and Families Who Changed Medicine Forever.* BenBella Books, 2020.

Weir, Peter, dir. *Dead Poets Society.* Touchstone Pictures, 1989.

Wilder, Thornton. *Our Town: A Play in Three Acts.* Harper Perennial Modern Classics. Reprinted 2003.

FOCOLARE MEDIA

Enkindling the Spirit of Unity

The New City Press book you are holding in your hands is one of the many resources produced by Focolare Media, which is a ministry of the Focolare Movement in North America. The Focolare is a worldwide community of people who feel called to bring about the realization of Jesus' prayer: "That all may be one" (see John 17:21).

Focolare Media wants to be your primary resource for connecting with people, ideas, and practices that build unity. Our mission is to provide content that empowers people to grow spiritually, improve relationships, engage in dialogue, and foster collaboration within the Church and throughout society.

Visit www.focolaremedia.com to learn more about all of New City Press's books, our award-winning magazine *Living City*, videos, podcasts, events, and free resources.

NCP
NEW CITY PRESS

www.ingramcontent.com/pod-product-compliance
Lightning Source LLC
Chambersburg PA
CBHW071049280326
41928CB00050B/2149